Read what others are saying about Your...

"*Sex and Your Heart Health* is a much-needed book. My experience in roles ranging from therapist and coach to family member and patient dealing with a health condition confirms that many of us patients are in desperate need of information that goes beyond general 'website information' about our disease or health condition. We don't want a medical degree, but we need specific information about how our bodies work; realistic information about how our disease or condition affects our body's functioning, our 'self' and our relationships; and practical strategies for living life with our condition. You provide this kind of information in a clear, easy-to-understand way. Thank you."

Lynne Hornyak, Ph.D., PCC
Editor and Author:
Experiential Therapies for Eating Disorders and
Healing From Within: The Use of Hypnosis in Women's
Health Care

"This book is just wonderful. It is down-to-earth and practical. I would definitely recommend it to my patients. It would be great for nurses and nursing students as well. It expresses complex ideas in a clear way. Physician assistants and medical students would also like it. I recommend it highly!"

Mary Havelka Martin, R.N.

"*Sex and Your Heart Health* is very easy to read and interesting. The authors have taken a complicated topic for the nonmedical person and made it very informative and enjoyable. Their book will be very helpful to many, including mental health professionals."

Jennifer L. Baker, PsyD, LMFT
Director, Marriage and Family Therapy Program
Forest Institute of Professional Psychology

"I think this book is really good! I especially like the areas where the authors talk about themselves. It gives readers a comfortable feeling like they actually know them—nice touch...This is a good read in easy-to-understand language."

Shelley White, Librarian

"The Stratmanns' book demystifies Cardiology. It would help anyone who is interested in the heart or in heart disease and wants to know more. It is really for everybody."

J.M., Heart Patient

Sex and Your Heart Health

Sex and Your Heart Health

A CARDIOLOGIST TELLS ALL

by

Henry G. Stratmann, M.D., F.A.C.C., F.A.C.P., F.C.C.P.

Maryellen Stratmann, M.D.

Nonfiction Division
Starship Press, LLC
Springfield, MO
www.sexandyourhearthealth.com

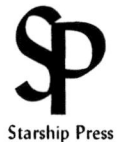

Starship Press

Sex and Your Heart Health
A Cardiologist Tells All

Copyright © 2007 by Henry G. Stratmann and Maryellen Stratmann

Manufactured in the United States of America

All rights reserved. No part of this book may be reproduced or used by any means including photocopying, graphic, mechanical, electronic, recording, storage in a database or information retrieval system, or otherwise without prior written permission from the authors, except by a reviewer or journalist, who may use brief passages in a review. For information, please contact Starship Press, LLC, 4319 S. National, #135, Springfield, MO 65810-2607 or through our web site at www.sexandyourhearthealth.com.

Notice: Medical knowledge and practice are continuously expanding and changing. The authors of this work have reviewed reliable sources of medical information and drawn on their own experiences as practicing physicians in writing this book. However, due to the possibility of human error and changes in medical care and treatment, neither the authors, the publisher, nor anyone else who has contributed to preparing or publishing this work warrants that the information within it is every way complete or accurate, and they disclaim any responsibility for any omissions, errors, or results associated with use of the information contained within this work. Readers are advised to consult their own physician or other health care professional regarding any questions about their health care and condition and how the information contained in this work might relate to their health. Internet addresses included in this book were accurate at the time this book was written.

Stratmann, Henry G. (Henry George)
    Sex and your heart health : a cardiologist tells all
/ Henry G. Stratmann and Maryellen Stratmann.
    p. cm.
    Includes index.
    LCCN 2006909126
    ISBN 0-9790480-0-1
    ISBN-13: 978-0-9790480-0-5

    1. Heart—Diseases. 2. Heart—Diseases—Patients—Sexual behavior. 3. Hygiene, Sexual. I. Stratmann, Maryellen. II. Title.

RC682.S785 2007   616.1'2
                                QBI06-200092

Published by
Nonfiction Division
Starship Press, LLC
4319 S. National, #135
Springfield, MO 65810-2607
www.sexandyourhearthealth.com

Printed in the United States by
Morris Publishing
3212 East Highway 30
Kearney, NE 68847
1-800-650-7888

INTRODUCTION

THIS BOOK IS for you—and you—and you!

Sex is one of God's greatest gifts to man and woman.

If you have heart disease, you might worry about having sex and not enjoy it as much as you should. This book is for you.

If you are fortunate enough to have a healthy heart, you want to continue leading a full life, living and loving well into your golden years. This book is also for you.

And if you are simply curious—well, this book is for you too!

Medical students, physician assistants, nurses, psychologists, clergy, marriage counselors, and other professionals will also benefit from this book. Heart disease remains the number one killer in America for both men and women. It touches everyone's lives.

The study of the heart and heart disease is one of the most complex areas of Medicine and one of the most difficult to master. We have distilled and condensed a massive amount of information and presented it in a conversational but frank manner.

This book was not written to be a cardiology textbook or exhaustive medical reference work on this topic. It was designed as a general introduction to sex and the heart and is based on our combined fifty-plus years of experience as physicians.

Use this book to gain a better understanding of sex and of your heart. Use it to become more comfortable talking to your own doctor about sex and your health. But do not let it substitute for advice from your own personal physician, who knows your particular situation best.

HGS and MES

ABOUT THE AUTHORS

From the Heartland of America

Henry G. Stratmann, M.D., F.A.C.C., F.A.C.P., F.C.C.P., is Clinical Professor of Medicine at St. Louis University in St. Louis, Missouri. He is board-certified in both Internal Medicine and in the specialty of Cardiovascular Disease.

A highly respected cardiologist for over 25 years, Henry is recognized as a superb clinician and a topnotch teacher. He has authored or co-authored over seventy peer-reviewed scientific publications.

Henry grew up raising chickens in a small town in southern Illinois. His down-to-earth upbringing is reflected in his practical approach to difficult topics.

Maryellen Stratmann, M.D., grew up in a blue-collar neighborhood in Cleveland, Ohio. She worked her way through medical school and graduated from Case Western Reserve University School of Medicine in 1981.

Maryellen did her internship and subsequent specialty training at Barnes Hospital and Washington University in St. Louis. She is board-certified in both Diagnostic Radiology and Nuclear Radiology. She has taught medical students and physicians in training from both St. Louis University and Washington University.

She is currently an Adjunct Professor at Drury University.

Maryellen and Henry have been married for over 22 years and have two teenage sons. They currently reside in the beautiful Ozarks in Missouri, the heartland of America. They both enjoy writing fiction and nonfiction.

Dedication

To our sons, Henry G. Stratmann III
and Joseph T. Stratmann.
Yes, boys, Mom and Dad really did have sex!

ACKNOWLEDGMENTS

WE, THE AUTHORS, wish to thank the medical school faculty at Southern Illinois University and Case Western Reserve University for starting us off on our careers. We also wish to thank the dedicated teachers we encountered during internship, residency, and fellowship training at St. Louis University (Henry) and at Washington University (Maryellen) in St. Louis. We are indebted to the "giants" in our fields who influenced us and stressed the quest for excellence.

We are particularly indebted to the nurses, doctors, psychologists, educators, and many others who reviewed all or part of our book.

Special thanks are extended to Dr. James Markusic, Mary Havelka Martin, Dr. Jennifer Baker, Tessa S. Melançon, Dr. Lynne Hornyak, Shelley White, Dr. Stephen Post, Jerry Maurer, and Dr. Stephen Bogdewic.

We also thank Heloise for calling to encourage us to get the word out about heart disease prevention, detection, and treatment. This gracious lady is a speaker and advocate for the American Heart Association.

In addition, we thank members of the Ozarks Romance Authors and Springfield Writers' Guild for their valuable support and suggestions.

We also thank Tom Davis for the interior text design. We are grateful to Ruth Hunter for the excellent job that she did designing the book cover.

Any mistakes that we have made are inadvertent and our own. We have done our best to share our knowledge about both sex and your heart health.

Preface

THE IDEA FOR *Sex and Your Heart Health* was conceived in our bedroom. Sometime during the afterglow, one of us murmured that sex was a lot more enjoyable way for married couples to keep their hearts in shape than dieting or working out at a fitness center. The conversation somehow turned to how people with heart disease could maintain a healthy, active sex life. Why, it might even make a good subject for a book! Soon we were laughing together at possible chapter titles like "Pills and Penises" and "Ventricles and Vaginas," as well as XXX-rated ones we'll leave to your imagination.

A bit later we realized that heart disease and sex really *was* a serious topic for a book. When a person has a heart attack or other serious heart problem, the doctor's first priority is to decide what tests and procedures need to be done and which medicines to give. At some point the doctor, nurse, or other health professional typically give instructions about diet, exercise, and any restrictions on activities at work or at home. However, a critical question that too often gets "lost in the shuffle" is whether or when it's safe to have sex. Too often the patient and spouse don't ask, and the doctor and nurse don't tell.

Sex and Your Heart Health is designed to help you learn about heart disease and how it may affect your sex life. It gives practical information on a wide variety of common and not so common heart problems. It tells how you can do your best to live with them or, much better, avoid developing them. Of course, everything we discuss is based on general ideas and facts. It's essential that you talk to your own doctor about any suspected or known heart problems you may have and how they impact your sex life.

Besides our combined fifty-plus years of professional experience as physicians, we also bring to *Sex and Your Heart Health* the pleasures and pains of over twenty-two years of marriage to each other. We are both doctors *and* spouses, sensitive to both the medical and personal impact heart disease may have on a couple's sex life. We hope the knowledge and feelings we bring from being both physicians and lovers come through in our book.

HGS and MES

Contents

Introduction vii

About the Authors ix

Dedication xi

Acknowledgments xiii

Preface xv

Chapter 1: Sex and More Sex! 23
   How Doctors Learn About Sex

Chapter 2: The Playful Pronk 27
   Anatomy and Function of Your Sex Organs
      Female Sexual Anatomy 29
      Male Sexual Anatomy 32
      Physiology and Hormones 36
      The Act of Sexual Intercourse 42
      Talking to Your Doctor About Sex 46

Chapter 3: Orgasm and Oxytocin 51
   Intimacy and Intercourse Issues
      Why Does Sex Exist? 52
      Unique Features of Human Sexuality 54
      Orgasm 55
      Oxytocin 57
      Intimacy Without Intercourse 58

Chapter 4: Getting Pumped 61
   Anatomy and Function of Your Heart
      Heart Chambers and Valves 62

Arteries and Veins 63
Pumps and Electricity 65
Blood Pressure 66
Coronary Arteries 67

Chapter 5: Size Matters 71
When Arteries Go Bad
    Coronary Artery Disease 72
    Heart Attacks 74
    Heart Failure 78
    High Blood Pressure 84
    Carotid, Aortic, and Peripheral Arterial
    Disease 85

Chapter 6: From Valves to Veins 95
Other Major Causes of Heart Problems
    Diseases of the Heart Valves 96
    Infective Endocarditis 100
    Heart Tumors 102
    Pericardial Disease 103
    Congenital Heart Disease 104
    Arrhythmias 105
    Deep Vein Thrombosis and Pulmonary
    Embolism 112

Chapter 7: Heart Attack! 115
Recognizing and Treating a Heart Attack
    Initial Treatment of a Heart Attack 117
    "Blood Thinners" for Heart Attacks 120
    Beta-blockers and Other Medications ... 121
    Arrhythmias and Heart Attacks 123
    Evaluation of Chest Pain 127
    Inside the Intensive Care Unit 131
    Thrombolytic Treatment and
    Coronary Angiography 133

Chapter 8: High-Tech Heart Tests 139
   Evaluating Risks to Your Heart
      Modern Stress Tests 140
      Echocardiography 142
      Myocardial Perfusion Imaging 146
      Pharmacologic Stress Testing 149
      Complications of a Heart Attack 151
      Home from the Hospital 154

Chapter 9: More Tests and Treatments 159
   Managing and Medicating Heart and
   Blood Vessel Disease 159
      At the Doctor's Office 160
      Tests for Arrhythmias 165
      Magnetic Resonance Imaging and
      Computed Tomography 167
      Tests for Arterial Disease 171
      Medications for Heart Disease 173
      Cardiology in the Future 183

Chapter 10: Mending a Broken Heart 187
   Procedures and Operations for the Heart
   and Blood Vessels
      Coronary Angioplasty 188
      Restenosis After Coronary Angioplasty .. 192
      Coronary Artery Bypass Surgery 195
      Transmyocardial Laser
      Revascularization 198
      Enhanced External Counterpulsation ... 199
      Artificial Heart Valves 201
      Surgery for Aortic Dissection and
      Aortic Aneurysms 207
      Surgery for Carotid and Other Arterial
      Disease 208

  Surgery for Congenital Heart Disease ... 208
  Cardiac Transplantation 210
  Mechanical Hearts 211
  Pacemakers and Implantable
  Cardioverter-Defibrillators 213

Chapter 11: Sex After Surgery 221
 From the Operating Room to the Bedroom
  Sex After Coronary Angiography 222
  Sex After a Pacemaker 223
  Sex After Heart Surgery 224

Chapter 12: Pills and Penises 231
 Medicines and Sexual Dysfunction in Men
  Erectile Dysfunction 232
  Beta-blockers and Sexual Dysfunction .. 233
  Other Heart Medications and Sexual
  Dysfunction 238
  Medications Used to Treat Sexual
  Dysfunction 240
  Other Treatments for Sexual
  Dysfunction 243
  Heart Disease and Sexual Dysfunction .. 245
  Evaluating the Safety of Sexual Activity . 246
  Assessing the Risk of Sex with Heart
  Disease 248

Chapter 13: Oh, Baby! 253
 Pregnancy and Heart Disease
  Pregnancy and the Normal Heart 255
  Pregnancy and Palpitations 256
  Peripartum Cardiomyopathy 258
  Pregnancy and High Blood Pressure 259
  Pregnancy and Coronary Artery Disease . 260

Pregnancy and Congenital Heart
Disease 262
Pregnancy and Severe Congenital Heart
Disease 264
Pregnancy and Pulmonary
Hypertension 264
Pregnancy and Myocarditis 268
Pregnancy and Arrhythmias 268
Pregnancy and Heart Valve Disease 269
Pregnancy and Artificial Heart Valves ... 271
Pregnancy and Heart Medications 272
Pregnancy and Warfarin 275
Pregnancy and Cardiac Testing 278

Chapter 14: Women and Heart Disease 281
When a Woman's Heart Breaks
Medications and Menopause 282
Birth Control Pills and Heart Disease ... 285
Medicines and Sex in Women 286
Women and Coronary Artery Disease ... 286
Evaluating Coronary Artery Disease
in Women 288
Treating Coronary Artery Disease
in Women 289
Women and Stroke 290
Women and Arrhythmias 291
Women and Heart Valve Disease 291
Women and Heart Failure 291

Chapter 15: Your Lifestyle and Your Love Life .. 295
Health Choices That Affect Your Sex Life
Diet and Heart Disease 297
Weight Loss 302
Exercise 304
Nutritional Supplements 306

Heart Disease and Alcohol 309
Tobacco and the Heart 309
Illegal Drugs 312
Health and Sex 314
Sex and Alcohol 315
Sex and Tobacco 316
Heart Disease and Sexually Transmitted
Diseases 317

Chapter 16: Spirituality, Psychology, and Sex ... 323
   Suggestions for Self-Help
      The Power of Prayer 324
      The Effect of Marriage on Heart Health .. 327
      Coping and Counseling 331
      Volunteer! 331
      Laughter and Loving 332
      Get a Hobby 334
      Age Doesn't Matter 334

Table 1. Common Symptoms and Treatments of
   Major Cardiovascular Diseases 337

Table 2. Major Types of Cardiovascular
   Medicines 341

Glossary and Definitions of Acronyms 345

References and Suggested Reading 353

Index 357

Chapter 1: Sex and More Sex!
How doctors learn about sex

Chapter Preview:
Medical Training and Sexuality
  Lectures and textbooks
  Educational movies
Experience
  Learning to be nonjudgmental
  On-the-job training

HAVE YOU EVER wondered how doctors learn about sex? No, we're not talking about the personal experience kind of learning. That varies a lot from doctor to doctor, just as with everyone else. What we're talking about is how sex and sexuality are taught in medical school.

Our medical school curriculum included courses in anatomy and physiology, the study of how the human body functions. But besides listening to dry lectures and reading scientific textbooks on the reproductive system, we were also shown movies of people having sex. Young couples and octogenarians. People with and without disabilities. People having sex with themselves. People having sex with partners of the opposite sex. People having sex with partners of the same sex. If there was an anatomically possible way for two or more people in various combinations of genders to physically couple, we studied how it was done. (We can just see applications to medical school booming once this becomes common knowledge.)

We both attended parochial grade school, high school, and college, and while we felt extremely well prepared for the academic side of medical school, we weren't prepared for this! However, 25 years later, we understand the wisdom of having been educated about a wide range of sexual expression. It also served as a kind of desensitization process. Know that you can speak to your doctor about sex without embarrassment, because he or she has truly seen it all!

Maryellen recalls one of her first stints working in the emergency room. A nurse handed her the X-ray of her next patient. Something that looked like a twelve-inch long metal rocket with battery parts stared back at her from the film. It was obviously lodged in the pelvis—in the vicinity of the rectum.

"It's a vibrator," the nurse said bluntly, "and he can't get it out."

It was the first of several "lost" vibrators that Maryellen would see in her future career as a radiologist. Interestingly, most of the patients claimed that they had accidentally sat on them! One of them told her, "I don't care if you can't get it out right away, just turn it off!" But another patient's mechanically assisted sexual encounter with himself turned out far worse. The vibrator tore a hole in his colon and he died.

Doctors are also taught to be nonjudgmental. Although we personally believe that sex should be reserved for a committed relationship between two loving people, we don't try to judge anyone or impose our own religious beliefs on them. Our job is to help you get well and to share ways to improve and maintain your health.

Television provides a skewed look at physicians. To attract viewers, doctors have been portrayed as having sex in the corridors, in the linen closets, and even in the elevators.

We have taken many hospital elevators over the years. Let us assure you that the only thing that goes "up" is the elevator!

Even if an intern wanted to "do it," medical ethics aside, the chances are that he or she would be much too tired. Fortunately, rules exist today that limit doctors in training from working more than 80 hours a week. However, when we began our medical education in the 1970s, we often worked in excess of 100 hours per week.

Not many people realize the number of years it takes to become a practicing physician. Usually, it's four years of college, four years of medical school, and a year of internship before you can even apply for a permanent medical license.

In addition to three years of internal medicine training after medical school, a cardiologist must also complete at least an additional three years of cardiology fellowship. This is usually followed by an extra one to two years of training in the cardiac catheterization suite and the noninvasive cardiology testing laboratory. Rigorous written exams must be passed along the way, including a final exam on cardiovascular disease.

About 15 or 16 years usually pass after high school before a cardiologist becomes "board-certified" in his or her specialty. Other types of physicians also have long training periods. Keep that in mind when you get your next doctor's bill!

Chapter 1 Summary

♥ Doctors learn about sexuality as part of their medical training. They are taught to be nonjudgmental.

♥ Share any sexual concerns you may have with your doctor or health care provider.

Chapter 2: The Playful Pronk
Anatomy and Function of Your Sex Organs

Chapter Preview:
Introductory Comments
    X and Y chromosomes
Female Sexual Anatomy
    Ovaries
    Uterus and cervix
    Vagina and clitoris
Male Sexual Anatomy
    Testes and scrotum
    Tube system for sperm transport
    Penis
Physiology and Hormones
    Gender and childhood
    Puberty
    Ovulation and menstruation
The Act of Sexual Intercourse
    Preparing for coitus
    Factors in achieving an erection
    Orgasm
    Contraception
Talking to Your Doctor About Sex

WE MET IN St. Louis after Henry placed a personal ad in the singles' section of a local newspaper, the *Riverfront Times*. Maryellen answered it on a dare from a friend. The ad cost $9.25. Since we are still happily married, we think it was a good investment.

If you decide to meet someone this way, we recommend you use the most extreme caution and meet in the daytime in a public place. We each drove our own cars to our first few meetings and Maryellen initially didn't give her address or her last name. We arranged to meet for the first time at 10:00 a.m. for Sunday Mass at Immacolata Catholic Church.

We spent part of our second date at the world-famous St. Louis Zoo, located in Forest Park in midtown St. Louis. Both of us enjoyed reading the plaques on the animal enclosures. Maryellen was enthralled by the lesser kudu and read aloud how they "pronked" in the brush and forests of east Africa. Although we later learned the word just meant they could leap high, the plaque made it sound like it was the technical term for how the male and female of the species made little lesser kudus. Maryellen liked the sound of the word pronk. After we were married, we liked to initiate lovemaking with each other by asking if we could pronk.

Such playful code words or inside jokes can definitely help a couple connect both emotionally and physically. However, when talking to your doctor it's better to use standard terms like "intercourse" or just "sex." After all, not everybody knows what "pronk" means! In this chapter we'll give a general overview of the biology of sex and the correct medical terms for the body parts involved.

Here's an interesting fact you may not know: before birth, at the time of conception, every baby starts out as a female. It takes a properly functioning Y chromosome stimulating production of male hormones like testosterone early in the baby's development to turn roughly half of all babies into males. The Y chromosome is by far the smallest of the twenty-three pairs of chromosomes in a human cell. This fact might make those of us of the male persuasion a bit more humble.

In any event, a male winds up with one Y chromosome and one X chromosome while a female has two X chromosomes. Except for this one important difference, men and women share the same total number of chromosomes in their cells—forty-six, with the two sex chromosomes (X and Y, or a pair of X chromosomes) joined by two each of the other twenty-two types of chromosomes. Rarely, a baby may be born with a different number of sex chromosomes. A female may have a single X chromosome (XO, Turner's syndrome), or a male may have an extra X chromosome (XXY, Klinefelter's syndrome). Individuals with these abnormal numbers of sex chromosomes have characteristic anatomic abnormalities and are infertile due to problems with the development of some of their sex organs.

Female Sexual Anatomy
Since a woman's sex organs really represent the prototype or "standard" for the human body, we'll start with a description of female anatomy. Two ovaries, each about an inch in length and shaped like an almond, are located on either side in a woman's pelvis (Figure 1, page 49). They are the main source for her sex hormones—estrogen, progesterone, and even a small amount of the male sex hormone, testosterone. The ovaries are also the source of all the eggs or ova that constitute her contribution to making a baby.

A single mature egg cell or ovum is about 1/250 of an inch in size. In its immature form, or "oocyte," the egg is located in a tiny fluid-filled space called a follicle along the walls of the ovary. About midway through her mother's pregnancy, a baby girl has up to seven million immature eggs in her ovaries. However, after reaching that peak number she will not produce any more eggs. The total number of immature egg cells will fall throughout the rest of her life due to her body breaking these eggs down and destroying them. By the time she's born, the number of eggs has decreased to about one to two million. By puberty she has about four hundred thousand left. The number of eggs continues to decrease as she matures until, with menopause, they are practically all gone.

A fallopian tube connects each ovary to the upper cavity of the uterus or womb. The uterus is a pear-shaped hollow organ with the stem end pointing downward. It is located just behind the bladder and in front of the rectum and is held in place by several ligaments. The uterus holds and nourishes the baby during a normal pregnancy. It is made of very stretchable muscular tissue that allows it to expand tremendously during pregnancy.

The inner lining of the uterus, the endometrium, contains specialized cells that nourish a fertilized egg after it implants itself into the uterus. Early during pregnancy, some of these endometrial cells form part of the placenta, an organ attached to the inner wall of the uterus. The placenta secretes progesterone and other hormones to help maintain the pregnancy. The mother and her developing baby are connected together by the umbilical cord, which forms by about the fifth week of pregnancy. This cord is attached to the placenta at one end and to the baby at his or her umbilicus or "belly button" at the other end. The umbilical cord usually contains two arteries and one vein. These blood vessels are surrounded by a spongy tissue that resists twisting and compression. Both the placenta and the umbilical cord supply the baby with blood, oxygen, and nutrients.

The uterus narrows down into a kind of spout called the cervix. Cervix is the Latin word for "neck," since this is the neck of the uterus. The cervix is shaped like a short thick cylinder with a small opening called the cervical os at one end. The inner walls of the cervix produce mucus. This mucus is usually thick and plugs the opening of the cervix. The mucus plug blocks fluids like semen from entering the uterus and helps prevent infection. However, as we'll discuss later, this mucus isn't always thick or a barrier to fluids passing through the cervix.

The cervix peeks partly into the upper vagina. The word vagina means "sheath," because this is the part of the woman's body that sheathes or encircles the penis while it slides in and out during sexual intercourse. The vagina is between four to five inches long and is composed of muscle tissue. The third of the vagina closest to the outside of a woman's body has a special elastic type of muscle that helps her control how wide its opening is. Normally the walls of the vagina are collapsed together, separating only during intercourse. The inner lining of the vagina has ridges called rugae and secretes fluid that, along with other secretions from glands around the cervix, keeps it moist.

Of course, the vagina leads to the outside of the woman's body. The vagina has an entrance called the introitus. In a girl or woman who's never had sexual intercourse the introitus is usually partially covered by a thin tissue called the hymen. Above the introitus is the separate and much smaller opening of the urethra (figure 2, page 49). The urethra is the tube that carries urine out of the body from the bladder.

Externally, above the urethra, is an important erectile organ, the clitoris. Its tissue has a rich supply of blood vessels and nerve fibers. The clitoris has about as many nerve endings as the penis. These nerve endings play the same role of providing pleasurable sensations in both organs. The tip of the clitoris, the glans, is at least partly covered by a small hood or prepuce. The clitoris also has an internal component. Running up and down on either side of the vagina's opening are two pink, relatively thin tissues called the labia minora—translated from Latin, the "little lips." Running parallel to them are two mounds of thicker tissue called the labia majora, or "big lips." The mons pubis is the small mound of tissue above the clitoris and vagina. In adult women, the mons pubis and labia majora are covered by pubic hair. This hair extends in an upside-down triangular pattern over the vulva, the name given to a woman's external genital area.

Male Sexual Anatomy
The differences between the sex organs of men and woman aren't as great as external appearances suggest. A man's sex organs are, for the most part, modifications of a woman's. The two testicles or testes ("testis" if you're talking about only one of them) started out as ovaries but changed due to the actions of the Y chromosome. Before birth the testes normally migrate down from the pelvis to ultimately take up permanent residence in the protective, bag-like scrotum. In about 3 to 4% of baby boys, one or both testes haven't yet made it down to the scrotum by the time they are born. However, most of these "undescended" testes will make it there within the first year of life. If a testis remains within the pelvis, a condition called cryptorchidism, this may not only decrease fertility in later life but also increases the chance of the undescended testis developing cancer. Imaging tests such as an ultrasound or a magnetic resonance imaging study can be used to locate an undescended testis.

The testes produce the male hormone testosterone and spermatozoa ("sperm" for short). Sperm cells are the man's contribution to baby making. These sperm cells are very tiny. In fact, a sperm cell is the smallest cell in the human body. In its mature form, a sperm cell consists of a microscopic head containing half the genetic material needed to conceive a baby; a narrow neck; and a proportionately very long whip-like tail that propels it through fluids in the man's body and, if it gets lucky, the woman's body too. Despite their small size, sperm cells are powerful swimmers. When active they can swim at a rate of about one-tenth of an inch every minute, whipping their tiny tails at a rate of about 200 times per minute. While the speed at which they swim may not seem very fast, when you take into account the sperm cell's size, it's the equivalent of a human swimmer going at a rate of over thirty-five feet per second!

It takes about seventy days for a sperm cell to develop from an immature form to a mature form. In a healthy adult male, each testis contains billions of sperm cells. A testis can produce millions of sperm each day for a total of twelve trillion or so over a man's entire lifetime.

The scrotum is the skin-covered pouch that holds the two testes. It forms from the same tissues that, without the influence of the Y chromosome and testosterone, would have formed the labia majora. The purpose of the scrotum is to house and protect the testes. True, the level of protection it provides is not very good during an altercation with someone who fights dirty. However, what the scrotum does well is to act as an air conditioning system for the testes. The scrotum keeps the testes about 4 degrees Fahrenheit cooler than they would have been if they had stayed within the pelvis. This is important because higher temperatures (like the classic 98.6 degrees Fahrenheit) inside the body itself reduce the number of sperm cells produced by the testes and increase the chance sperm will be abnormal. These effects would, of course, reduce a man's fertility.

Each testis hangs down within the scrotum like a ball (so to speak) on a rope. The rope-like structure each testis is attached to is called the spermatic cord. Each testis gets its blood supply through its own cord. Since the left spermatic cord is usually longer than the right, the left testis often hangs down a little lower than the one on the right. This information will hopefully reassure all you men who've wondered since your teenage years if there was something "wrong" with you down there—no, it's perfectly normal.

A muscle that is part of each spermatic cord, the cremasteric muscle, acts as an additional temperature-regulation system. The cremasteric muscles contract when a man is cold, bringing the testes closer to the warmth of the inner body. This helps the testes maintain their normal temperature. When a man is warm these muscles relax and the testes move away from that same internal heat source. Each cremasteric muscle also contracts and raises the testis attached to it when a man's upper inner thigh is stroked near the scrotum—the cremasteric reflex— or when he is under stress.

A series of tubes and structures with still more fancy names—seminiferous tubules, seminal vesicles, epididymis, and vas deferens—act as a plumbing system that allows sperm cells to move from the testes and out of the body. Sperm cells originate in the seminiferous tubules within the testes. These sperm cells then move through a series of tiny tubes ("efferent ducts") to a storage area adjacent to each testis called the epididymis (Figure 3, page 50). When sperm cells are mature, they pass through additional ducts to the vas deferens, another tubular structure that acts as a storage and transport area.

The vas deferens feeds into the urethra near where the urethra inserts into the bladder. The urethra is significantly longer in men than in women. In a man it courses from the bladder, through the prostate gland, and then via the penis to the outside of a man's body. The spermatic fluid (semen) that ultimately passes into the urethra consists primarily of fluid secreted by the prostate gland and the seminal vesicles—small glands that sit behind the bladder and above the prostate. Sperm cells actually make up only about 5% of semen. Both urine and spermatic fluid can travel through the urethra. A small sphincter—a ring of muscle that can tighten and relax—located where the urethra enters the bladder normally prevents this from happening at the same time.

The urethra is surrounded by the penis. The penis is—literally—a "clitoris on steroids." Testosterone and other male sex hormones are all members of a class of chemicals our bodies produce naturally called steroids. While a developing baby boy is still in his mother's womb, these natural "anabolic steroids" turn what would have been a woman's small (but mighty!) erectile organ, the clitoris, into a man's considerably larger organ, the penis.

The shaft of the penis consists of columns or cylinders made up of important tissues. In the center, surrounding the urethra, is the "corpus spongiosum." Adjacent to the corpus spongiosum is erectile tissue called the "corpus cavernosum." Just below the skin of the penis is fibrous tissue called the "tunica albuginea." At the end of penis is the glans or, less formally, its head. In Latin, glans means "acorn"—and it does look a bit like one, doesn't it? The foreskin is the thin tissue that covers the penis when it is relaxed. The foreskin retracts, exposing the glans of the penis, when a man has an erection.

Physiology and Hormones
In short, each gender's basic anatomy develops before birth in response to our body's hormones. During childhood, the same sex hormones that make us male or female in our mother's womb take a back seat. Children produce only very small amounts of sex hormones. However, sometime late in childhood the pituitary gland in the brain begins to secrete increasing amounts of substances called luteinizing hormone and follicle-stimulating hormone. Luteinizing hormone causes the ovaries and testes to start producing large amounts of sex hormones, while follicle-stimulating hormone is needed for production of mature egg and sperm cells. As these hormone levels rise, puberty begins.

Puberty is when "secondary" sex changes occur—some cosmetic, others essential to actually using our sex organs. As boys turn into men, voices deepen; hair develops on the face, chest, underarms, and groin; muscles get proportionately larger; and bones grow faster, leading to a "growth spurt" and increased height. Most importantly, the penis and testes enlarge and the sperm needed to produce offspring start to be made. All this is in response to the surge in testosterone production that occurs early in puberty.

All these changes occur over a period of at least several years. The average age they start in boys is somewhere between 9 and 14, with an increase in size of the testes and, about a year later, enlargement of the penis being the first signs of things to come. (Sorry about that!) Growth of pubic hair, growth of hair on other parts of the body like the face and chest, lowering of the voice, and other physical changes occur over the next several years. Toward the end of puberty, males acquire the ability to have a full erection and ejaculate. This can happen normally during sleep—a "nocturnal emission" or, less technically, a "wet dream."

For girls, puberty can begin as early as 6 years old, with the breasts starting to enlarge. Most changes, however, start later, usually between ages 8 and 13. As with boys, hair grows on the underarms, legs, and pubic area, and the genitals assume their mature appearance. Besides growing in height and weight, girls also normally develop increased fat in the buttocks, belly, and legs.

The most dramatic change in girls is the start of their menstrual cycles. The first menstrual period (menarche) usually occurs between ages 10 and 16, with an average age of about 12. While girls have had immature eggs in their ovaries from birth, at least one egg now matures each month and is capable of being fertilized. The normal menstrual cycle occurs over a period of about twenty-eight days, give or take a week.

At the beginning of the menstrual cycle, a rise in blood levels of follicle-stimulating hormone stimulates up to seven oocytes (immature eggs) to each start developing into a mature egg cell (ovum). Each ovum is protected inside a tiny fluid-filled capsule called a follicle. Only one of these follicles and the ovum inside it usually reaches full maturity during each cycle. Its unsuccessful competitors wither away and die. If two of them do make it to maturity around the time of sexual intercourse, however, one ovum can be fertilized by one sperm cell and the other ovum fertilized by a different sperm cell. This results in nonidentical twins. Identical twins are caused by a single fertilized egg dividing in two.

The mature follicle produces estrogens that change the lining of the uterus (the endometrium) so that, if a fertilized egg reaches it at the right time, the egg can attach itself and grow there. By about day 12 of the menstrual cycle, the follicle is large enough to form a small bulge on the ovary. The follicle also triggers the pituitary gland to secrete more luteinizing hormone for the next several days. This causes the follicle to release the ovum itself into the fallopian tube—"ovulation." The ovum then slowly migrates through the fallopian tube to the uterus.

During ovulation, in the middle part of their menstrual cycle, women may experience pelvic pain or discomfort called *mittelschmerz*. Sometimes this pain is so severe it can mimic appendicitis and lead to a visit to the emergency room, where a computed tomography (CT) scan or other imaging test might be done to sort out what is causing the pain.

As we've discussed before, the cervix produces mucus that is usually thick and forms a plug that blocks fluids from entering the cervix. However, around the time of ovulation, the mucus becomes thin and the cervix releases its "mucus plug." Women may notice secretion of this stringy mucus from the vagina. With their path no longer blocked by this mucus plug, sperm cells are now able to enter the cervix and swim through the rest of the uterus into the fallopian tubes where fertilization of the ovum can occur.

During ejaculation, a man produces only about a teaspoonful of semen. This fluid contains up to about five hundred million sperm cells. Their journey through the vagina, cervix, and body of the uterus is so long and hazardous, however, that by the time they reach the opening to each fallopian tube the number of sperm cells has diminished to as low as the hundreds.

Usually only one of the fallopian tubes contains a waiting ovum, so many of these sperm cells will choose wrong and wind up in a dead end. Of the ones that enter the correct fallopian tube (maybe, unlike the typical man, they actually do ask for directions!), only the fastest and luckiest sperm cell finally bumps into the ovum. The sperm cell's head penetrates the ovum, its tail falls off—and the union of the sperm cell and ovum starts a new baby. The fertilized egg then continues its journey toward the uterus.

Rarely, the fertilized egg doesn't make it to the uterus, and the baby starts to grow in the fallopian tube itself. This "ectopic" or "tubal" pregnancy occurs in about 1 to 2% of pregnancies. An ectopic pregnancy can present as a life-threatening surgical emergency. Early in the pregnancy, the mother experiences lower abdominal pain due to the tube being stretched by the growing baby. Unlike the uterus, the fallopian tube is simply not made to hold a growing baby. Eventually the fallopian tube can rupture, causing bleeding and potentially death for the mother. Much more rarely the fertilized egg can wind up somewhere else outside the uterus, such as within the ovary or the abdomen (belly) itself.

While the mother with an ectopic pregnancy can be helped, except in very rare cases, the developing baby itself cannot be saved. The baby may be destroyed spontaneously by the mother's body, or it may need to be removed by surgery or by using certain medicines like methotrexate.

A newly fertilized egg is called a "zygote." About four days after conception, when the zygote begins to divide into more cells, the growing baby is then called an "embryo." By eight weeks after conception, most of the baby's organs have formed or are developing. From that time on, until he or she is born, the baby is called a "fetus."

Whether or not fertilization occurs, the now empty follicle changes into the "corpus luteum" (Latin for "yellow body"). The corpus luteum can grow to be even larger than the ovary itself—over two inches in diameter. The corpus luteum secretes both estrogen and progesterone for about the next two weeks, during the second half of the menstrual cycle. These hormones further prepare the uterus to accept a fertilized egg. If fertilization and implantation—that is, attachment of the fertilized egg to the inner wall of the uterus—does occur, the woman's body produces a new substance, human chorionic gonadotropin (HCG). Standard pregnancy tests measure if the woman has an elevated level of HCG. This chemical gives the rest of the body and the corpus luteum the message, "Baby on board!" The corpus luteum then continues to secrete progesterone, which is needed to sustain the pregnancy.

The ovum has about a 24-hour deadline to be fertilized or not. If, as usually happens, the ovum isn't fertilized, it is destroyed. The corpus luteum doesn't get the signal to keep on producing progesterone and degenerates into an area of scar tissue called the "corpus albicans." Progesterone levels fall, signaling the uterus, "No baby this month!" Since the tissue lining the inner wall of the uterus that was waiting for the fertilized egg isn't needed, this tissue sloughs off. In most animals, the female merely breaks down and absorbs this material. However, in humans and some other primates, a mixture of this tissue and blood flows out of her body through the vagina—"menstruation."

The average amount of blood a woman loses each month with menstruation is about one to three ounces—enough to potentially cause a mild anemia (low blood count). After an average of three to five days of bleeding, the menstrual cycle starts all over again, repeating every month unless pregnancy or menopause occurs. Menopause is reached when a woman hasn't had a menstrual period for one year. This usually occurs between ages 45 and 55. For several years prior to menopause, menstrual cycles typically becoming irregular. During this time, the ovaries produce less estrogen and progesterone. The number of oocytes in the ovaries drops dramatically, ovulation stops, and the woman can no longer become pregnant—at least by the conventional method.

For several years prior to menopause, a "premenopausal" woman may have symptoms that include hot flashes or flushes, irritability, sudden episodes of sweating (especially at night), problems sleeping, and weight gain. Not all of these symptoms occur in every woman or occur to the same degree. As we'll discuss in Chapter 14, hormone replacement therapy with estrogen and progesterone can relieve some of these symptoms, such as hot flashes.

Unlike women, whose stores of egg cells fall continuously from the moment they're born and are eventually lost, men normally produce new sperm cells throughout their entire lives. They do not experience the dramatic changes in sexual function women do in middle age. However, as they age, men do generally have a more gradual decrease in sexual interest and performance. This so-called "andropause" (the "andro" part is based on the Greek word for man and the term "androgens," the general name given to male sex hormones like testosterone) is usually subtler than menopause is in women. Andropause can be associated with difficulty achieving and sustaining an erection, lower sperm counts, and loss of interest in sex. Nonetheless, unlike women, who lose their fertility at menopause, it is possible for a healthy man to father a child (though with decreasing odds of success) well into his Medicare years.

The Act of Sexual Intercourse

Now let's put all this information about male and female anatomy together (so to speak). Engaging in sexual intercourse—the technical term is "coitus"—requires the presence and proper functioning of all the anatomy we've just discussed. In women it begins with thinking sexual thoughts, physical contact such as hugging or kissing with her partner, and direct stimulation of the genitalia, breasts, or other sensitive parts of her body. This foreplay activates certain parts of the brain and the nerves, primarily the pudendal nerve and sacral plexus, that connect her genital organs with her spinal cord.

Parasympathetic nerves in particular are important for preparing the woman for intercourse. These nerves dilate (widen) the arteries in erectile tissues (like the clitoris) and stimulate secretion of fluid into the vagina. This fluid is produced by glands near the cervix and by the walls of the vagina itself. The fluid acts as a natural lubricant. It produces a massaging rather than irritating effect on both the vagina and the penis and helps both partners achieve climax.

Before the penis enters the vagina, however, it must be able to achieve an erection. This results from a complex interplay between the vascular and nervous systems that supply the penis. Through a process similar to what happens in a woman, sexual thoughts and physical stimulation cause parasympathetic impulses to pass from the sacral spinal cord through the pelvic nerves to the penis. This makes the penile arteries and the smooth muscle in its erectile tissue (the corpora cavernosum we talked about earlier) relax. The latter contains large cavernous sinusoids (hollow spaces) that normally are nearly empty of blood. These sinusoids dilate tremendously when arterial blood flows into them under pressure and the flow of venous blood out of them is partially blocked. Since this erectile tissue is surrounded by the strong fibrous tissue of the tunica albuginea, when all this extra blood rushes into the penis and can't get out easily, the net effect is hardening, rising, and elongation of the penis. If the man hasn't been circumcised, the foreskin also retracts from the glans of the penis.

Once the penis is firm enough for penetration, the partners can assume any of a variety of positions that allow the penis to move parallel to the walls of the vagina. Before or at the time of penetration, the muscles at the woman's introitus relax to allow the penis to enter. Once inside the vagina, it's critical that the penis doesn't get "bent" too much. If the partners are in a position that allows one or both to make a sudden shift in the wrong direction, the medical term for what might happen next is a "penile fracture"—and yes, it is just as bad as it sounds. For example, this can happen when the woman is in the superior position, the penis slips out of the vagina, and she accidentally brings her full weight down and "straightens" the penis towards its nonerect direction.

This very unfortunate turn of events can cause a "cracking" sound, followed in very short order by excruciating pain, bleeding, swelling, and deformity of the penis. These problems are caused by a tear in the fibrous tissue within the penis. Surgery is usually needed to repair the injured organ—and, of course, further (hopefully more cautious) attempts at intercourse aren't an option until the penis has healed.

Assuming that things have gone smoothly, however, stimulation of the penis and clitoris causes an orgasm (climax) in one or (hopefully) both partners. Orgasm requires stimulation from nerve impulses originating in the spinal cord and the sympathetic nervous system. In the man, orgasm leads to a series of contractions in the ducts and organs that carry sperm and seminal fluid, as well as contractions in the bulbocavernosus muscle at the base of the penis. These contractions ejaculate semen out through the urethra and into the vagina.

Immediately after orgasm and ejaculation, its duty done, the penis loses its erection. For a highly variable time afterwards measured in minutes to hours, the penis temporarily cannot be stimulated to regain an erection. Eventually, over another highly variable period, it becomes "partially refractory"—able to become "sort of" erect and possibly capable of another orgasm. Finally, after enough time has passed, full function does return. As many wives have observed, while waiting for this to happen the man's natural biological response may be to roll over and go to sleep.

However, this "natural" male response is unlikely to be prudent or perhaps even safe for him due to his wife's reactions to his post-lovemaking drowsiness. Women generally become sexually stimulated more slowly than men but stay stimulated longer. Moreover, they have the distinct advantage over men of not being limited to the typical "one orgasm and you're done." During lovemaking, women are capable of many and frequent orgasms with no discernible refractory period between them. From a strictly biological standpoint, it's essential that the man has an orgasm during intercourse for the woman to become pregnant, but it is not an absolute necessity that she has one (or more). From a practical standpoint, however, whether or not pregnancy is the goal of a particular sexual encounter, it's a good thing for both partners to feel sexually satisfied. If that means the man has to defer his nap until his wife feels equally satisfied, so be it.

Whether or not pregnancy occurs after intercourse depends on where the woman is in her menstrual cycle and whether she and her husband have used any form of contraception or birth control prior to or during intercourse. The moral implications of artificial methods of birth control are outside the scope of this book.

Temporary types of contraception include, in roughly decreasing order of effectiveness, various combinations of estrogen with or without progesterone-like chemicals called "progestins" that suppress the menstrual cycle, used in the form of pills, injections, implants, patches, or vaginal rings; intrauterine devices (IUDs); barrier methods, including condoms, the vaginal diaphragm, and cervical cap, all of which may be used with spermicidal material; early withdrawal of the penis from the vagina before ejaculation ("coitus interruptus"); and "rhythm" or "natural family planning" (NFP) methods based on having intercourse when the woman is least likely to be fertile during her menstrual cycle.

Permanent forms of birth control include tubal sterilization in the woman, which involves blocking off or cutting the fallopian tubes so sperm can't reach the egg, and vasectomy in the man, in which the tubes leading from the vas deferens are blocked so sperm can't get into the semen.

There are two controversial methods of birth control that can be used shortly after sexual intercourse has already occurred. One method involves a woman taking a large dose of a progestin either by itself or with estrogen within seventy-two hours after sexual intercourse. Levonorgestrel ("Plan B") is a progestin that is thought to work primarily by suppressing ovulation so that a mature ovum isn't released and fertilized. A second method is to place an IUD, particularly one containing copper, as soon as possible after sexual intercourse. The IUD is thought to work by destroying sperm cells and egg cells. The major controversy with both of these methods is that they might also prevent a fertilized egg from implanting itself in the uterus, causing the egg's destruction.

If none of these methods of birth control is used and two fertile partners have unprotected sex, pregnancy can occur if a woman is at or near the ovulation phase of her menstrual cycle. Besides the limited time the mature ovum produced during ovulation is available for fertilization, the other major factor as to whether pregnancy results is exactly when sperm are "introduced" into the vagina. Sperm cells can survive for only a few hours in the open air if they are ejaculated onto skin or another external surface rather than into the vagina. However, if these sperm cells reach the cervix and enter the uterus or a fallopian tube, they can survive for up to about five days. This means that having intercourse several days before the woman actually ovulates can still potentially result in pregnancy.

Talking to Your Doctor About Sex
Human sexuality is a very complex topic and goes far beyond the basic anatomy and physiology we've

discussed here. While doctors routinely talk about all these subjects in a purely matter-of-fact way (OK, maybe not 100% of the time—if you're married to another physician!), our patients sometimes seem embarrassed when it comes to talking about sex. They may also be vague or use slang terms for their sexual organs. When Maryellen was working in the Pediatric department, a mother brought her daughter into the clinic, saying her daughter's "monkey" was hurting. Maryellen wondered if they were really looking for the veterinarian's office until it dawned on her that the "monkey" meant her daughter's external genital area.

When talking to your physician, it's best to use the standard medical terms for sex organs that we just reviewed. Doctors say them as easily as they say "wrist" or "ankle." Practice saying "vagina" and "penis" out loud at home, though not necessarily in front of your kids or the repairman who comes to fix your refrigerator. Your doctor will try to make you as comfortable as possible when you do.

Chapter 2 Summary

- ♥ In a female, the ovaries produce egg cells and sex hormones such as estrogen and progesterone.

- ♥ In a male, the testes produce sperm cells and the sex hormone testosterone.

- ♥ Intercourse requires a complex interplay involving multiple body systems, including the endocrine system, the cardiovascular system, and the nervous system.

♥ The possibility of sexually transmitted diseases and pregnancy occurring should be considered before a couple has sex.

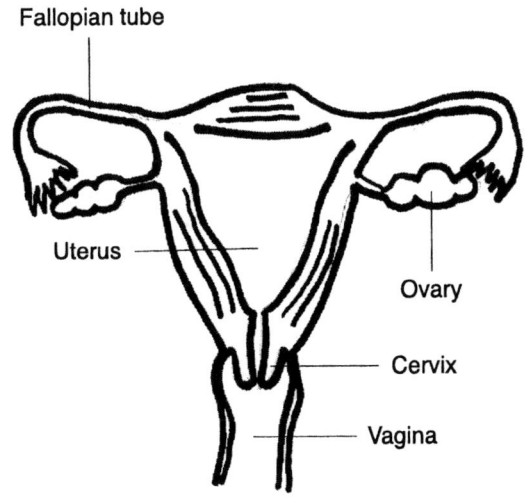

Figure 1. Internal female anatomy, simplified and not to scale, as seen from the front (coronal view).

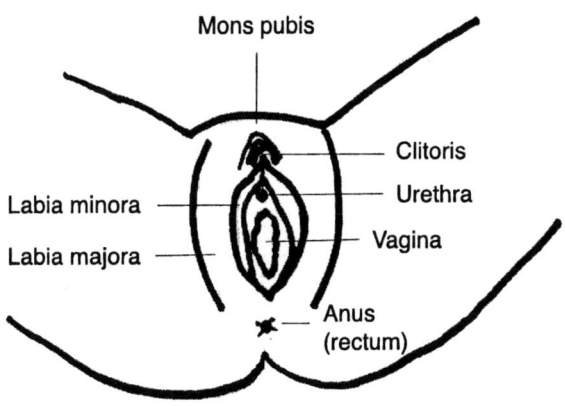

Figure 2. External female anatomy, simplified and not to scale, as seen from between the legs (lithotomy position).

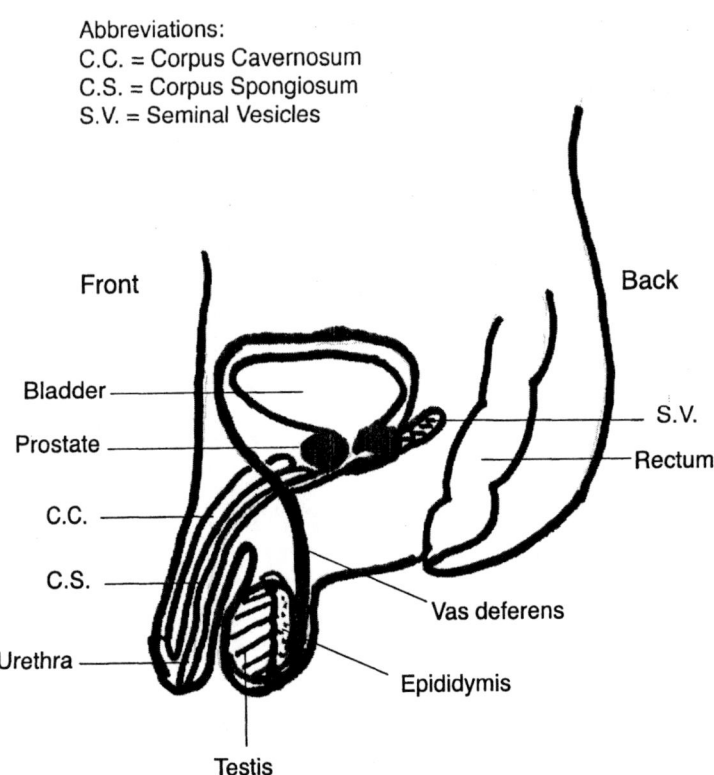

Figure 3. Male internal and external anatomy, simplified and not drawn to scale, as seen from the side (sagittal view).

Chapter 3: Orgasm and Oxytocin
Intimacy and Intercourse Issues

Chapter Preview:
Why Does Sex Exist?
    Asexual versus sexual reproduction
    Survival of the species
Unique Features of Human Sexuality
    Self-awareness
    Availability for sex
    Other considerations
Orgasm
    Psychological and physical factors
    Body and brain links
Oxytocin
    Biological roles
    Psychological roles
Intimacy Without Intercourse
    Medical and moral considerations
    Love as biochemistry
    Love as a decision

DO YOU KNOW that the English word "sex" is based on the Bible? "Sex" is Latin for the number six. In the Ten Commandments of the Old Testament, it is the sixth commandment—"Thou shalt not commit adultery"—that has to do with sex.

When we use the word "sex" in this book, we are referring to sex in the Biblical sense, that is, the act of sexual intercourse. Let's face it. It was faster and easier for us to type "sex" instead of "intercourse" or its really fancy name "coitus" every time we used the term. In addition, we also use the word "sex" to refer to our gender as a man or a woman. A person's gender has both physical and psychological implications.

Why Does Sex Exist?

The most basic biologic function of sex in humans or any other animal is reproduction. Individual members of a species eventually die due to disease, accidents, predators, or old age. New, young individuals must replace the old for a species to continue.

A few simple animals such as sea anemones, sponges, and flatworms can reproduce either without sex (asexually) or by sexual reproduction. Other animals, such as earthworms, leeches, or certain types of fish like sea bass can either change during their life cycle from male to female (or vice versa) or be both simultaneously. However, mammals and nearly all other vertebrates (animals with a backbone) must permanently develop into one or the other gender for successful reproduction.

Asexual reproduction has the obvious advantage that no "help" is necessary for an animal to reproduce. Cut off the arm of a starfish or split off part of a flatworm and a complete new individual can grow from that severed portion. This new animal is a true "clone," genetically identical to its parent. Asexual reproduction also works well for animals like sea anemones that aren't always mobile. Sea anemones often attach themselves to a rock and stay there for a long time—drastically reducing their chances of finding a mate. Budding a new individual off their body solves this problem. Asexual reproduction can also be used to produce many offspring in a short time.

However, asexual reproduction has a major disadvantage. Since offspring are genetically identical to the parent, a new disease or a stressful change in their environment means they will all be equally vulnerable to it.

Sexual reproduction results in "genetic diversity." Each offspring shares some, but not all, characteristics of its parents. It is a new combination of different genetic material obtained from each parent. Now if a new disease develops or living conditions worsen, some of the species' offspring will be more vulnerable or likely to die than their parents. Others will have about the same risk. But some offspring will be more likely to survive. These latter individuals will be most likely to reproduce and pass on these same characteristics to their offspring. This process of "natural selection" increases the odds that a species as a whole will survive a change in its environment.

This major advantage of sexual reproduction compared to the asexual variety helps explain why this is the only way mammals reproduce *naturally*. Another reason is that mammals consist of many more highly specialized cells than simple animals like a sea anemone. The cells in muscle, nerves, and other parts of the body can't on their own change to a form that could grow into a new mammal. Some mammals can be cloned—a form of asexual reproduction. However, this requires highly artificial, nonnatural techniques. Otherwise, with the exception of identical twins, every baby mammal is genetically unique.

Human beings are mammals. We share the same basic biological reason for having sex as other animals do. Like aardvarks and anteaters, bears and bison, we *Homo sapiens* need to have enough of us produce offspring for our species to survive. Like other mammals, our brains and bodies are "programmed" with an instinct and drive to have sex.

With one exception, every organ system in your body—your heart, lungs, digestive system, etc.—is needed to keep you alive and healthy. That exception is your reproductive system. There's an absolute need for every person to breathe, eat, and eliminate waste. By comparison, sexual activity is optional. It is not *absolutely* required for an individual to stay alive. Sexual reproduction is needed only for a *species* to survive. Enough of its members must successfully reproduce for the species to continue. However, it is *not* necessary for any *particular* individual to have sex.

However, this isn't the whole story.

Unique Features of Human Sexuality

Humans have two major differences from other mammals that make sex a much more complicated affair than this. We humans are animals, but we are *self-aware* animals. Although we have instincts like other animals, we have the potential to understand our actions and the freedom to make choices as to what we do.

Humans and several other primates (including chimpanzees, gorillas, and orangutans) also differ with nearly all other mammals in another important way. In these other mammals sex is seasonal—that is, sex occurs only at specific times. Instead of a menstrual cycle, females of these other species have an "estrous cycle." Sex generally occurs only during one phase of this cycle—the "estrus" phase, when the female is "in heat." This is when her eggs are either ready to be fertilized or, as in cats and some other animals, the production of eggs that can be fertilized is actually caused by sexual intercourse.

Thus, in these other animals, sex is intermittent. There are long periods of time with little or no sexual activity. Roughly the opposite state of affairs occurs in humans. We can *choose* to be sexually active or not at any time with a willing partner. This element of choice means that having sex involves much more than other biological processes such as eating food or having a bowel movement.

Because intercourse can result in sexually transmitted diseases (STDs), monogamy is the most medically beneficial choice for human beings. It is estimated that STDs affect over 65 million Americans. Some STDs, such as gonorrhea or chlamydia, can be cured with proper treatment. Others, like genital herpes and the human immunodeficiency virus (HIV, the virus that causes AIDS—"acquired immune deficiency syndrome"), can be treated but *not* cured. STDs may have other implications as well. Human papillomavirus is an STD that increases risk of cervical cancer in women. A new vaccine can help prevent it. However, there is no cure for the millions of women already infected. Some STDs can lead to infertility. Some, such as syphilis and HIV, can be transmitted from an infected mother to her baby.

Because sexual intercourse can also result in offspring, and because it is a deep emotional and psychological as well as physical experience, we also feel that sex is best performed in the context of a long-term committed relationship.

Orgasm

In the prior chapter we discussed the physical act of sexual intercourse. Here, we'll focus on orgasm, the term that refers to sexual climax. Orgasm results in feelings of relaxation and release.

Orgasm involves "vasocongestion" (increased blood flow) to the lower pelvis and sexual structures. It is accompanied by muscle contractions in the pelvis, especially the muscles involving our sex organs and anal region. There may also be muscle contractions, spasm, or rigidity in various parts of the remainder of the body. Orgasm involves interplay between our psyche and multiple organ systems, including the endocrine system, the circulatory system, the nervous system, and the musculoskeletal system.

Men can have orgasm without ejaculation or even ejaculation without orgasm, although usually they happen together. Orgasm does not always occur with intercourse in women. In fact, it has been reported in some scientific studies that as few as 30% of women achieve orgasm from the act of sexual intercourse. To have an orgasm during intercourse, the woman or her partner usually must stimulate her clitoris. Less frequently, orgasm can result from vaginal stimulation, stimulation of the breasts or other parts of her body, and even from thoughts.

Especially in women, orgasm occurs due to a complex interplay of physical factors, psychological factors, and relationship factors. Illness, injury to the pelvic area, certain medications, and prior surgery can all interfere with orgasm. Anxiety and fear may also shift blood flow away from the sex organs and prevent orgasm from occurring. Depression can decrease desire and also interfere with orgasm and other aspects of sexual function. The effect of antidepressants and other medications is well known and will be discussed in a separate chapter.

Besides changes in the rest of the body, orgasm is accompanied by changes in the brain. Orgasm has been described on positron-emission tomography (PET) as causing decreased activity or function in the amygdala region of the brain.

An important substance called oxytocin is also released into the bloodstream during orgasm.

Oxytocin
Oxytocin is a hormone and a neurotransmitter (a chemical that helps messages pass between nerve cells). This hormone is made within the brain by the hypothalamus. Oxytocin is then stored and secreted from the posterior pituitary gland at the base of the brain.

The amount of oxytocin in the blood increases in pregnant women during labor. Oxytocin causes contractions of the uterus that help the baby to be born. Oxytocin is also involved in lactation—ejection of milk from the mother's breasts. In addition, oxytocin helps a mother to bond with her infant.

Our understanding of oxytocin and all the things that it does continues to grow. Oxytocin is released from both men and women at orgasm. Our blood levels of oxytocin may increase three to five times above normal during orgasm. Oxytocin increases bonding or feelings of attachment between sexual partners. This effect may be more pronounced in women than in men.

Oxytocin is also thought to counteract stress. It decreases blood pressure and helps to lower anxiety levels. Oxytocin has a calming effect. It may promote healing or recovery from illness and may increase pain thresholds. Oxytocin may be partly responsible for married people living longer than unmarried people.

Touch itself may also cause oxytocin to be released, particularly in women. Oxytocin in turn may promote the desire to touch and be touched in a kind of feedback loop.

While adrenaline (epinephrine) is known as the "fight or flight" hormone, oxytocin has been called the "tend and befriend" and the "cuddle" hormone. Oxytocin is involved with social behaviors and may be involved in the formation of trust.

Oxytocin also has so-called "amnestic" properties. That means it may help us forget an incident that hurt us. This may be beneficial to couples when they "kiss and make up" after an argument.

Intimacy Without Intercourse
There are many situations in life when we cannot have sexual intercourse even if we are married and have a willing partner. These situations might include a medical illness, when complications occur during pregnancy, following certain kinds of surgery, and during the first six weeks or so after childbirth.

An individual also may not choose to have sex outside of marriage due to religious, philosophical, or moral beliefs. It is important to honor those beliefs and not pressure him or her.

We spoke with James Markusic, Ph.D., a psychotherapist and adjunct professor at Drury University. Dr. Markusic is a popular professor within the educational community and has been honored by Drury as an "Educator of the Year." He is often sought out for consultation.

"Feelings of guilt and other psychological difficulties may result if individuals engage in sex against their belief system," explains Dr. Markusic. "This can occur not only in young people, but in older couples as well. As individuals and as a society, we must recognize and respect this. We need to teach the difference between sex and love."

When a couple initially falls in love, biochemicals including phenylethylamine (PEA), dopamine, and norepinephrine come into play. These substances contribute to the giddy, walking-on-air feeling people get when they fall in love. Eventually the "high" these chemicals give us wears off. This may take months to a year or perhaps a little longer to happen. While these chemicals can certainly make a person feel good, they can also cloud judgment and make it difficult to make sound decisions regarding sex.

We like to think of true love as a decision rather than only a fleeting feeling or a chemical response. We are not always in control of our feelings. However, as human beings, we should be in control of and responsible for our decisions.

Sometimes not having sex is a greater act of love than having sex. For example, your partner may be just "too tired" or too preoccupied with something that is worrying him or her to desire or enjoy a sexual encounter. Also, you may not always have the privacy that you need. These times are opportunities to explore other ways of expressing physical love and affection. Hugging, kissing, a massage, caressing, or simply holding each other are all ways to show that you care.

Intimacy does not have to mean only sexual intercourse. Some of our most intimate moments as a couple occurred at times in our life story when we could not express genital sex for various reasons.

"In fact," says psychotherapist Dr. Markusic, "lovers of all ages should learn alternate ways to express intimacy besides sexual intercourse. These alternate ways may be more appropriate for their career and life goals, as well as their overall value system. How we express our sexuality has tremendous implications for lifestyle and personhood and is also crucial for developing and maintaining a sense of self-worth."

Love can be expressed in many ways. Performing acts of service for each other, such as helping with household chores or driving the kids to school, and showing appreciation to your partner are also important ways to express love. These actions may also involve oxytocin. Regardless of the biochemistry behind these acts of love, a couple will still reap practical benefits from them today and in times to come.

Chapter 3 Summary

- ♥ Sex is necessary for the survival of our species but not for the survival of any one individual.

- ♥ Unlike other animals, human beings can decide when or if to have sex.

- ♥ Physical, psychological, and relationship factors are involved in achieving orgasm. Oxytocin is released during orgasm and helps partners bond.

- ♥ Love and intimacy can also be expressed without intercourse.

Chapter 4: Getting Pumped
Anatomy and Function of Your Heart

Chapter Preview:
Heart Chambers and Valves
   Atria and ventricles
   Heart valves
Arteries and Veins
   The right-sided heart pump
   The left-sided heart pump
   Carbon dioxide and oxygen exchange
Pumps and Electricity
   Systole and diastole
   Electrical impulses in the heart
Blood Pressure
   Systolic blood pressure
   Diastolic blood pressure
Coronary Arteries
   The three major coronary arteries
   Variations in size and supply

YOUR HEART NEVER gets a day off from work. You can rest your weary bones and muscles in an easy chair and let your brain slip into a nap. If your body would let you do it, you could even safely shut down your liver, your kidneys, your pancreas, and one lung (not both, please!) for several hours or more. But your heart can never stop working.

When you're born your heart is thumping away at up to about 200 beats per minute. The average heart rate gradually slows down during childhood, settling down in adults to a mellow level of about 60 to 100 beats per minute when you're sitting quietly.

By the time you reach your thirtieth birthday your heart has beat at least two billion times—not even counting the times it's raced faster during exercise, excitement, and, of course, sex. And if you're reading this book, your heart is still working.

The normal heart weighs about ten to twelve ounces in an average-sized man and weighs several ounces less than that in a woman. Your heart sits behind your breastbone (sternum) and the third, fourth, and fifth ribs on the left side of your chest.

Heart Chambers and Valves

The heart has four chambers in humans and other mammals (Figure 4, page 70). The two upper, smaller chambers are the right atrium and the left atrium. They sit side by side, separated from each other by a shared wall called the interatrial septum. The two lower chambers, the right ventricle and the left ventricle, are larger and have thicker walls than the two atria. These two ventricles do most of the heart's work. Like the atria they sit side-by-side, completely separated from each other by the interventricular septum.

The heart has four valves—specialized flaps of tissue that allow blood to flow only one way through the heart. The tricuspid valve is located between the right atrium and the right ventricle. The pulmonic valve lies between the right ventricle and the pulmonary artery, the main blood vessel that sends blood to your lungs. The pulmonary artery divides into two major branches. The right pulmonary artery carries blood to your right lung, and the left pulmonary artery sends blood to your left lung. The mitral valve separates the left atrium from the left ventricle. The aortic valve regulates blood flow between the left ventricle and the aorta. The aorta is the large blood vessel that carries blood out of your heart to the rest of your body.

Arteries and Veins
Basically the heart is an electric-powered pump whose function is to keep blood circulating. More correctly, it's two pumps working together. The right atrium and right ventricle act together as one pump, while the left atrium and left ventricle form the second pump. When an atrium or ventricle fills with blood the special muscle in its walls contracts, squeezing blood forward into the next chamber or into a major blood vessel. Arteries and veins are the "pipes" that carry this blood throughout the body.

Turn your right hand so the palm is facing you. See those bluish streaks on your arm near your wrist? Those veins are carrying blood that's already run a race through your body and is heading toward the finish line in your right atrium. The blood is blue and "deoxygenated" because the cells in your brain, stomach, vagina or penis, etc. have already pulled out from it the oxygen they need to live and function. Hemoglobin, the chemical in your blood cells that carries oxygen, turns blue when the amount of oxygen it has on board drops below a certain level. Of course, when hemoglobin does pick up more oxygen in the lungs, it turns bright red—but we'll get to that later. Your body's cells exchange the oxygen they get from blood with another gas, carbon dioxide, which they produce as a waste product by merely being alive.

While carbon dioxide is perfectly fine for fizzy bubbles in soda or champagne, having too much of it in your blood is not healthy. Your heart and lungs work together to get rid of excess carbon dioxide and restore oxygen to your blood. That process begins once the blood in your veins reaches the right atrium. From there it flows into the right ventricle, which contracts and pumps blood into the pulmonary artery. This blood then goes through the lungs, eventually traveling through tiny blood vessels called capillaries.

In the capillaries of the lung, carbon dioxide is exchanged for more oxygen and your blood turns red again. Once out of the lungs this "rejuvenated" blood enters the left atrium through the pulmonary veins. The pulmonary veins are the only veins in the body that carry bright-red oxygenated blood. The blood flows from the left atrium into the left ventricle, where it is pumped into the aorta and out to the rest of the body.

At first the aorta heads in the direction of your head, but then it makes a U-turn down toward your legs. The aorta's overall shape is like a cane. The handle of the cane is made of the short "ascending" aorta, followed by another short section shaped like an inverted "U," the aortic arch. The long straight portion of the cane is the "descending aorta." Smaller arteries branching off of the aorta supply blood to your brain, arms, stomach, liver, spleen, and other internal organs.

At about the level of your belly button (the technical term is "umbilicus") the aorta splits into two arteries called the right and left iliac arteries. Branches of the iliac arteries supply your reproductive and sexual organs, including the clitoris and vagina if you're a woman and the penis if you're a man.

Eventually the red oxygenated blood in all of these arteries winds up in tiny capillaries throughout all of your organs. These organs extract oxygen from the blood in the capillaries, and then this blue deoxygenated blood enters your veins. This "venous" blood then makes its way back to your right atrium, where the entire process of "circulation" of the blood is repeated. On average, the left ventricle pumps out about four to six quarts of blood every minute in an adult who's sitting quietly. The amount of blood pumped out each minute—the "cardiac output"—increases when a person is more active.

Pumps and Electricity

All this flowing and pumping of blood has to occur in the right sequence and with the right timing to work. Both the right ventricle and the left ventricle contract at about the same time, during a part of their pumping cycle called "systole." The pressure created by the contracting right ventricle closes the tricuspid valve and opens the pulmonic valve so that blood flows only in the direction it should, into the pulmonary artery. Something similar is happening on the left side of the heart, where the left ventricle's contraction closes the mitral valve and opens the aortic valve, sending blood forward only into the aorta.

Once the two ventricles finish contracting, the pulmonic and aortic valves close and the tricuspid and mitral valves open. During "diastole," the second major part of the heart's cycle of filling and contracting, blood at first flows passively from the right atrium to the right ventricle and from the left atrium to the left ventricle. When the two ventricles have mostly filled with blood, the two atria normally contract to force an extra amount of blood into them (the so-called "atrial kick"). Once enough blood is in them, the ventricles contract, systole begins—and the cycle starts over again.

Getting the atria and ventricles to fill with blood and contract at the right times is the job of the heart's electrical system. Each of the four chambers of the heart needs an electrical impulse to make it contract. The sinus node, a small area of specialized cells located in the upper right corner of the right atrium, acts as the "ignition system" for the heart. The sinus node generates an electrical impulse that is carried by special fibers in the atria and ventricles. These fibers act as the heart's "wiring system." To make sure the ventricles don't get their electric signal to contract too soon, a special area of cells near the junction of the right atrium and right ventricle—the atrioventricular (AV) node—acts as a "speed bump." The AV node slows the electrical impulse created by the sinus node long enough to ensure the ventricles don't contract before the atria have filled them with a good supply of blood to pump.

Blood Pressure
Your blood pressure is the pressure in your aorta and other arteries generated by the pumping action of the left ventricle. The first number of the blood pressure, the systolic blood pressure, is the pressure in these arteries when the left ventricle is contracting. It normally runs about 100 to 130 millimeters of mercury (abbreviated mm Hg) when a person is sitting quietly. A systolic blood pressure between 90 to 100 mm Hg is borderline low. As systolic blood pressure drops below 90 mm Hg, it becomes increasingly likely a person will become lightheaded or even pass out due to the brain not getting enough blood. Systolic blood pressure normally goes up when a person exercises or is under stress. How much it goes up depends on how vigorous the exercise is.

The second number, the diastolic blood pressure, is the pressure in the aorta when the left ventricle isn't contracting and the aortic valve is closed. Normal range for this is about 60 to 80 mm Hg. Diastolic blood pressure may be lower than this, however, without causing any problems. The diastolic blood pressure usually stays the same or goes down a bit with exercise.

Coronary Arteries

Like every other part of the body, the heart also needs to be supplied with blood containing oxygen and nutrients. The very first arteries that come off of the aorta, just above the aortic valve, are the right and left coronary arteries. These two arteries supply blood to the heart itself.

The right coronary artery is usually the main source of blood for the right ventricle and the bottom (inferior) wall of the left ventricle. Just after it comes off the aorta, the left coronary artery has a very short segment called the "left main artery." The left main artery then quickly divides into two major branches. One branch, the left anterior descending artery, supplies blood to the front of the left ventricle (anterior wall and septum) and also usually provides blood to the apex (the end or "tip" of the heart). The other major branch of the left coronary artery, the circumflex artery, provides blood to the left side ("lateral wall") of the left ventricle.

The heart starts out with two coronary arteries, the right coronary artery and the left coronary artery. However, because the two major branches of the left coronary artery, the left anterior descending artery and the circumflex artery, are so large, these two arteries are considered coronary arteries in their own right. Thus, for practical purposes we have three coronary arteries—the right coronary artery, the left anterior descending artery, and the circumflex artery. Smaller branches of these three coronary arteries supply blood to specific areas of the heart. Once again, this arterial blood eventually winds up in capillaries and then in veins in the heart itself that feed back into the right atrium.

When it comes to the coronary arteries, one size does not fit all. There are many minor differences from one person to another regarding how large each of these coronary arteries is and, to some degree, what parts of the heart they supply. Except in uncommon cases, like a coronary artery originating from an abnormal location, as long as enough blood gets to where it's needed it doesn't make much difference exactly which artery supplies which part of the heart.

Overall this system of pumps and pipes does a great job of supplying blood, oxygen, and nutrients to the body. However, just as with the pipes, plumbing, and electrical system in your home, sometimes things break down. In the next chapter we'll discuss the major things that can go wrong with your heart and its blood vessels.

Chapter 4 Summary

- ♥ Think of the heart as a right-sided pump (right atrium and right ventricle) and a left-sided pump (left atrium and left ventricle).

- ♥ The right-sided pump carries venous blood to the lungs to replenish the blood's oxygen supply.

- ♥ The left-sided pump delivers blood replenished with oxygen from the lungs to the rest of the body.

♥ Three major coronary arteries supply blood to the heart muscle itself.

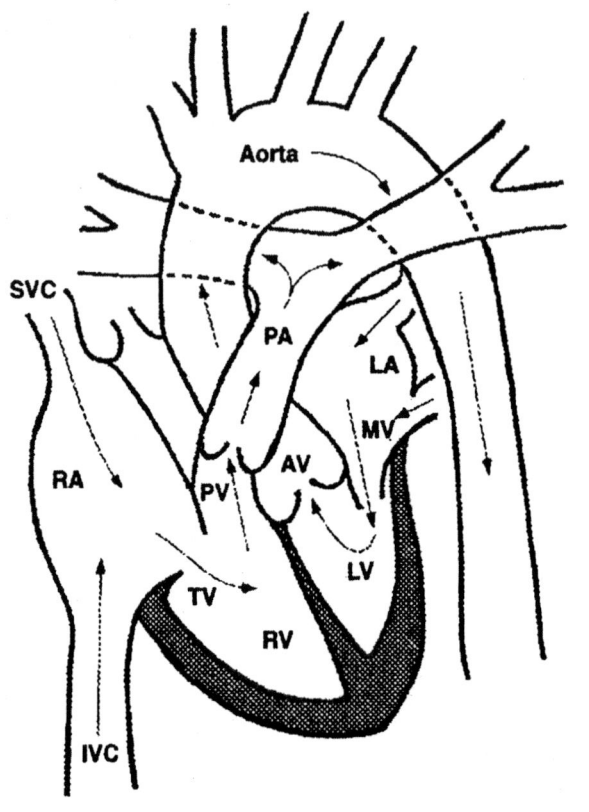

Chambers and valves of the heart. Arrows show direction of blood flow.
AV = aortic valve; **IVC** = inferior vena cava; **LA** = left atrium; **LV** = left ventricle; **MV** = mitral valve; **PA** = pulmonary artery; **PV** = pulmonic valve; **RA** = right atrium; **RV** = right ventricle; **SVC** = superior vena cava; **TV** = tricuspid valve.

Figure 4. Cardiac anatomy.

Chapter 5: Size Matters
When Arteries Go Bad

Chapter Preview:
Coronary Artery Disease
    Statistics
    Causative factors
    Significance
Heart Attacks
    Definition
    Causes
    Symptoms
Heart Failure
    Definition and statistics
    Types and causes
    Symptoms
High Blood Pressure
    Definition and prevalence
    Complications
Carotid, Aortic, and Peripheral Arterial Disease
    Aortic arch and its branches
    Transient ischemic attacks and strokes
    Aortic aneurysms
    Aortic dissection
    Arterial disease of the legs
    Risk factors

IN THE LAST chapter, we described what happens when the heart and its blood vessels are working the way they should. In this chapter, we'll talk about major ways this complicated system of pumps and pipes can go wrong. In later chapters, we'll discuss the medications, procedures, and other treatments used to fix what goes wrong with the heart and blood vessels.

Coronary Artery Disease

Coronary artery disease (CAD) is the name given to blockages that occur in the arteries of the heart. CAD kills more people in the United States each year than any other disease. It affects about thirteen million Americans and kills one of them every minute. The risks of an adult developing or dying from CAD increase with increasing age. The chance of developing CAD after age 40 is about 50% in men and 30% in women.

CAD is caused by "atherosclerosis." This disease is produced by injury to the inner lining (intima) of the coronary arteries. Raised areas of "atherosclerotic" plaque form inside the coronary arteries due to this injury to the intima. High blood pressure, elevated cholesterol, diabetes, and smoking are major causes for this injury and development of atherosclerosis. Atherosclerotic plaques start out as yellowish, fatty streaks on the intima. These fatty streaks can be present as early as age 10. Over time, damage to the coronary artery worsens due to inflammation and abnormal accumulation of muscle cells and cells containing fat ("foam cells") within the intima.

The most advanced stage of atherosclerosis is the fibrous plaque—a white, raised area that at least partly blocks off the artery itself. These plaques are usually fairly soft. As we'll see in later chapters, one treatment for these plaques is to compress them and make them smaller. However, especially in older people and those with diabetes, atherosclerotic plaques can also accumulate calcium and become hard and rock-like.

Blockages that involve more than 50% of the artery's diameter can reduce blood flow enough that heart muscle—"myocardium"— doesn't always get as much oxygen as it needs. This condition is called "myocardial ischemia." Myocardial ischemia can cause a type of chest pain called "angina pectoris" (Latin for "chest pain"). Angina is typically "substernal"—that is, the chest pain is felt under the breastbone. Angina is usually described as a pressure or sensation of a weight on the chest rather than an actual pain. The chest pain may spread into nearby parts of the body like the neck or the left shoulder and arm.

Angina may be accompanied by other symptoms, such as shortness of breath or sweating. Occasionally it may be felt in unusual ways, like a sensation of heartburn in the area of the body just below the breastbone. A person having myocardial ischemia may not even have angina or any symptoms at all—"silent ischemia."

Coronary blockages more than 50% but less than 90% typically cause angina only during exertion or when a person is under stress. Angina usually lasts no more than about five to ten minutes continuously. It usually goes away when a person stops exercising and rests. This is due to the heart needing more blood and oxygen when it's working harder than the blocked artery can supply. However, when the person is resting and the heart doesn't need as much blood and oxygen, the partially blocked artery can supply enough blood to the heart.

When a coronary artery blockage is 90% or more, however, the amount of blood getting to the area of the heart the artery supplies is less than normal even when a person is resting. A person with such a severe blockage may have angina not only with exertion but even when sitting or sleeping. Sometimes very small arteries called "collaterals" can develop between and connect a coronary artery with severe blockage and another coronary artery without severe blockage. These collaterals can help supply at least a little more blood to an area of the heart supplied by the coronary artery with the severe blockage.

Angina is considered "stable" when it occurs predictably (a person knows a certain amount of exertion will produce it), isn't occurring more frequently or with less exertion than before, and hasn't started to occur when a person isn't doing anything or is asleep. "Unstable" angina can include the first ever episode of angina. However, it more commonly refers to the pains becoming more frequent, severe, or occurring with less or no exertion.

CAD can involve one, two, or all three coronary arteries. It can occur in any part of the arteries. However, blockages due to CAD are more likely to occur in certain locations in the coronary arteries, such as where an artery branches off into smaller ones. While "obstructive" CAD (one or more blockages more than 50%) can cause myocardial ischemia and the symptoms we've described, people with "nonobstructive" CAD (one or more blockages 50% or less) are also at risk for serious problems. Over time these blockages can worsen and produce symptoms. Even more importantly, these milder, nonobstructive blockages are more likely to cause a heart attack than more severe blockages.

A wide variety of medications, procedures, and operations can now be used to treat CAD. We'll be discussing them in later chapters.

Heart Attacks
A heart attack ("myocardial infarction") occurs when a coronary artery becomes so severely blocked that it can't supply enough blood to an area of the heart to keep it alive. The typical way this happens is that a

blood clot suddenly forms on one of these atherosclerotic plaques, dramatically increasing the amount of blockage in the artery and often completely blocking it off. This blood clot formation can occur for many reasons, including rupture of the plaque or other injury to the area (such as that caused by smoking). Mild, nonobstructive blockages are generally more vulnerable to rupture of their atherosclerotic plaque and sudden formation of blood clots on them than more severe blockages are. This is why these milder blockages are generally more likely to cause a heart attack than tighter blockages.

Although a heart attack can occur during heavy exertion or severe stress, it is far more likely to happen when a person is doing only light activity, resting, or even just sleeping. This is because the most common causes of a heart attack, like plaque rupture, are not significantly related to whether or not a person is doing anything strenuous at the time.

In case you were wondering, the risk of having a heart attack during sex, either in men without known heart disease or those with heart disease considered to be at low risk, is very small. Less than 1% of heart attacks occur during sex. A healthy middle-aged man's risk of having a heart attack during or within two hours after sex has been reported to be about one to two out of a million. A healthy woman's risk having a heart attack during sex isn't as well known, but it would likely be about the same or lower.

In fact, some studies have shown that men who have more frequent sex are, overall, less likely to have heart attacks than less sexually active men! This may be partly due to the fact that sex requires a mild to moderate level of exercise. By having sex these men are "conditioning" their bodies to about the same degree as walking at a moderate pace for around fifteen minutes would do. It's fair to say that, given a choice of ways to exercise, most men would choose sex over a brisk walk on the treadmill!

Although the overall risk is still low, people with known heart disease and those who have significant risk factors for heart disease are at greater danger for a heart attack during sex than those who are healthy. In a later chapter we'll go into more detail about what types of heart problems increase this risk.

A person having a heart attack will typically have angina and other symptoms such as shortness of breath, sweating, nausea, lightheadedness, and the classic "sense of impending doom." However, unlike the typical episode of chest pain that lasts five to ten minutes, this pain lasts considerably longer. Chest pain usually continues as long as the artery is blocked or until the area of the heart the artery supplies dies. If the blood supply to the heart isn't restored within about twenty-five minutes, the area of the heart deprived of blood will begin to suffer some degree of damage.

A person can also have a "silent" heart attack, without chest pain or other symptoms. The chance of having a silent heart attack is higher in people with diabetes. This is because diabetes can reduce the ability of nerves to carry the sensation of pain. Other people may have symptoms that they don't recognize as being a heart attack. These "atypical" symptoms include shortness of breath or, especially with heart attacks involving the lower part of the heart, a sensation of heartburn rather than angina. It's more common for women and elderly people to have symptoms that might be due to other problems besides a heart attack, like shortness of breath or nausea, and not "classic" angina.

At the other end of the scale, all too often the most obvious sign that a person is having a heart attack is that the unfortunate individual collapses and dies suddenly. This occurs in about a third of people who have a heart attack. By far the most common reason for this is that, when an area of the heart is starved for blood, it not only causes pain and doesn't work as well but the heart's electrical system also goes haywire. These hurting heart cells generate electrical impulses that cause an abnormal, very fast heart rhythm. One of these fast heart rhythms, ventricular tachycardia, is caused by electrical impulses coming from one of the ventricles at a faster rate than the ones from the place they normally come from, the sinus node. Ventricular tachycardia can cause a heart rate as low as 110 beats per minute. At that heart rate, a person usually has only mild or no symptoms. However, ventricular tachycardia can go as fast as 400 beats per minute or more—too fast for blood to move in and out of the heart to supply the rest of the body.

A heart attack can also cause an even deadlier heart rhythm, ventricular fibrillation. With ventricular fibrillation, a ventricle is producing impulses that are so frequent and chaotic that the ventricle winds up just "quivering" with no effective pumping action at all. If ventricular fibrillation or very fast ventricular tachycardia isn't treated within minutes, the person will die due to lack of blood to the brain and the rest of the body.

In the next chapter we'll go into detail about how heart attacks are treated. Now we'll move on to another very common heart problem—heart failure.

Heart Failure

Heart failure occurs when the heart can't pump enough blood to meet the needs of the rest of the body. Heart failure is a very common heart problem, particularly as people get older. About five million Americans have heart failure. In both men and women, the risk of developing heart failure after age 40 is about one in five. In people diagnosed with heart failure before age 65, 70% of women and 80% of men will die within eight years. The risk of death is highest within the first year after heart failure is diagnosed—about 20%.

Heart failure is most commonly due to either weakness (systolic dysfunction) or increased stiffness (diastolic dysfunction) of the left ventricle. Many people can have both types of problems.

There are many different causes—some temporary, some permanent—for the left ventricle to become weak and not pump as well as it should. Let's briefly discuss some of the most common causes.

A heart attack can damage part of the left ventricle or, less commonly, the right ventricle. If the undamaged parts can't increase how much work they do to compensate for this damage, overall heart function decreases.

High blood pressure puts strain on the left ventricle over a long period of time. The left ventricle initially responds by increasing the thickness of its walls (left ventricular hypertrophy). Eventually, if high blood pressure isn't treated and controlled, the left ventricle may start to fail. It can become larger and pump less strongly.

Heart valve problems, particularly abnormal narrowing or leakage of the mitral or aortic valves, can also overwork the left ventricle and lead to heart failure. We'll talk about the major types of heart valve problems in a later chapter.

Infection and inflammation of the heart muscle—"myocarditis"—is usually caused by a viral infection. Myocarditis can cause either temporary or permanent weakness of the left ventricle as well as the other heart chambers. Certain medications and chronic use of too much alcohol can do the same thing.

Diabetics are at increased risk of developing heart failure. This is partly due to their increased chance of having CAD in large and medium-sized coronary arteries. As we've discussed before, this can cause a heart attack and damage the heart. But diabetics can also develop blockages in the tiniest arteries of the heart. This problem doesn't lead to a single big heart attack. Instead, it damages the heart a little at a time. As the blockage in each of these tiny arteries gets worse, the very small area of heart muscle it supplies with blood dies and forms scar tissue. Over time, if enough of these tiny arteries become diseased, large areas of the heart can be damaged and heart function decreases.

When a healthy person is sitting quietly the left ventricle pumps out about 50% to 65% of the blood inside it with each beat. This percentage of blood is called the "ejection fraction." People whose left ventricular systolic function and ejection fraction have fallen below normal may develop symptoms such as shortness of breath and fatigue. Their risk of having potentially life-threatening arrhythmias, such as ventricular tachycardia or ventricular fibrillation, also increases when left ventricular systolic function becomes moderately to severely reduced. People diagnosed with heart failure have an overall risk of "sudden death" (usually caused by these abnormal heart rhythms) that is about six to nine times higher than in the general population.

The chance of having symptoms or sudden death is generally quite small when the left ventricular ejection fraction is only mildly decreased to between 40% and 50%. However, the likelihood of having symptoms or sudden death begins to increase significantly once ejection fraction falls below 35% to 40%. People who are discovered to have an ejection fraction that is less than 20% have a particularly high risk of death. However, the risk of death in people with moderately or severely reduced left ventricular ejection fraction can be significantly reduced using certain medications and procedures we'll discuss in later chapters.

Heart failure can also occur when the amount of blood pumped out with each beat is either normal or more than normal, but the walls of the left ventricle are stiffer than usual. The left ventricle doesn't relax as much as it should to allow blood to come into it during diastole. As people age, this "diastolic dysfunction" becomes increasingly common. Anything that stimulates the walls of the left ventricle to become thicker and stiffer, like high blood pressure or severe aortic stenosis, can also do this.

One specific cause of diastolic dysfunction is hypertrophic obstructive cardiomyopathy (HOCM). This disease can run in families and is also referred to as "idiopathic hypertrophic subaortic stenosis." In HOCM certain parts of the left ventricle, particularly the interventricular septum, become abnormally thick—in some cases nearly twice the normal thickness. The abnormally thick septum causes partial blockage of blood flow out of the heart at a level right before the aortic valve. In these patients, the left ventricle may be contracting with either normal or increased strength, but this "subaortic" blockage prevents enough blood from getting out of the heart to the rest of the body. In fact, this blockage increases if either the left ventricle contracts more vigorously or if a person's heart rate increases. HOCM can also be associated with significant leaking of the mitral valve, abnormal heart rhythms, and eventual weakening of the left ventricle.

Many symptoms of heart failure are due to pressures in the left ventricle rising above normal. This occurs both with systolic dysfunction (weakness of the left ventricle) and with diastolic dysfunction (increased stiffness of the left ventricle). During diastole, when the left ventricle is filling with blood, the pressure inside it is transmitted back through the left atrium to the blood vessels of the lung (pulmonary vessels). If the pressure in the left ventricle becomes abnormally high due to weakness or increased stiffness of its walls, this pressure is transmitted back to the pulmonary vessels. If the pressure in these vessels becomes high enough, fluid will leak out of them into the lungs. This fluid replaces the air that is supposed to be in the lungs and causes shortness of breath.

Increased pressure in the pulmonary vessels will, in turn, be transmitted back to the right atrium and right ventricle. Eventually the right ventricle may enlarge and weaken from having to pump blood against this higher than normal pressure in the pulmonary blood vessels. Increased pressures in the right side of the heart are then transmitted back to the veins in the rest of the body. This can make fluid leak out of those veins and cause swelling of the legs (edema) and belly (ascites).

Shortness of breath, edema, and ascites are common symptoms associated with "congestive heart failure" (CHF). A person with mild CHF may become short of breath only when he tries to do something. Someone with more severe CHF may have trouble breathing even when he is just sitting still. He may also wake up at night short of breath. More blood from the veins in the legs comes back to the heart when a person is lying flat than when he is standing. This "extra" blood may be too much for a weakened heart to handle and makes more fluid slowly leak out into the lungs. Anywhere from minutes to several hours after going to bed, the person wakes up short of breath—"paroxysmal nocturnal dyspnea." Sitting on the side of the bed for a while or perhaps sleeping upright in a chair for the rest of the night usually helps him breathe easier. Propping his head and upper chest up on two or three pillows when he goes to bed can help prevent this breathing problem from occurring.

If the left ventricle can't pump enough blood, the rest of the body—brain, kidneys, muscles, etc.—also suffers. Heart failure can cause weakness and fatigue. If heart function isn't good enough to maintain a normal blood pressure, a person can become light-headed or even pass out (syncope). This is most likely to occur when a person who's lying down suddenly stands up. If the kidneys don't get enough blood they will react inappropriately by making the body retain salt and water. This can make the person gain weight and increase the amount of fluid leaking out into the lungs and legs. This fluid retention can be reduced by mildly restricting the amount of salt a person uses.

Another cause of heart failure, "high output" heart failure, is less common than that caused by systolic or diastolic dysfunction. In high output heart failure the heart itself is typically normal, but it can't supply enough blood to the body due to problems outside the heart. For example, a person with severe anemia may not have enough red blood cells to carry oxygen to the body's tissues even though the heart is contracting harder than normal. In hyperthyroidism, a gland located in the front of your neck, the thyroid gland, releases too much of a hormone called thyroxine into the bloodstream. Thyroxine stimulates many parts of the body, including the heart, and increases the amount of work they do and the amount of oxygen they need. In a person with hyperthyroidism, although the heart may be contracting harder and faster than normal, it still may not be able to meet the rest of the body's increased need for blood and oxygen. Other causes of high output heart failure include severe infection caused by bacteria in the blood (sepsis), beriberi (a disease caused by lack of vitamin B_1, thiamine), and abnormal blood flow between arteries and veins seen in certain conditions like Paget's disease (a disease of bone).

There are now many ways to treat heart failure using medications and operations. Heart failure caused by weakness of the left ventricle can be treated with medicines that improve the heart's ability to pump blood. These medications can both relieve symptoms of heart failure and decrease a person's risk of death. People with CAD may have an area of myocardium that is not getting enough blood to contract well, but the amount of blood is enough to prevent the myocardium from dying. This "hibernating myocardium" can eventually contract well again if its blood supply is restored by procedures such as coronary angioplasty or coronary artery bypass surgery. Severely damaged heart valves causing heart failure can be replaced to improve heart function. A heart transplant may also be an option in some people with severely weakened hearts.

We'll discuss the specific medications, procedures, and operations used to treat heart failure in later chapters.

High Blood Pressure

High blood pressure—hypertension—is defined as systolic blood pressure that is consistently 140 millimeters of mercury (mm Hg) or higher or diastolic blood pressure that is 90 mm Hg or greater. "Prehypertension" is defined as an average systolic blood pressure of 120 to 139 mm Hg or a diastolic blood pressure between 80 to 89 mm Hg.

These numbers are used to decide if a person has hypertension based the assumption that he or she is resting quietly. Systolic blood pressure normally goes above 140 mm Hg with exercise or stress. Therefore, blood pressure measurements should be taken after a person has been sitting quietly for about five minutes. Blood pressure also normally varies a great deal during the day. It is helpful for a person to measure blood pressure at home at different times of day for several weeks and record these readings in a small notebook. Your doctor can review the notebook to see if and how often your blood pressure is higher or lower than normal.

Stress and anxiety caused just by seeing your doctor can make the first blood pressure measured at your doctor's office higher than it normally is—"white coat hypertension." A second blood pressure measurement taken after you've relaxed may be significantly lower than the first one. If your blood pressure is only mildly above normal on a particular visit, your doctor may check it again on another visit or two to confirm it is consistently elevated before diagnosing you as having hypertension.

Hypertension is present in about one third of adults. It increases a person's risk of developing CAD, heart failure, kidney failure, and especially stroke. It is called the "silent killer" because, until a person develops these kinds of complications from it, hypertension usually causes no symptoms. Hypertension can even be seen in children, but it becomes more common as a person gets older. African-Americans have, on average, both a higher prevalence of hypertension and greater average blood pressure measurements than other Americans.

In about nine out of ten people hypertension is due to the body's own failure to regulate blood pressure well. This can be due to a person's arteries becoming stiffer as he gets older, inappropriate constriction ("clamping down") of the arteries, or the body retaining too much salt and water. Only about one out of ten cases of hypertension have a specific cause, such as kidney disease, blockage in the arteries of the kidneys, tumors, or medications like birth control pills.

Many medications are now available to treat hypertension (see Tables 1 and 2). It is common for a person to need two or more blood pressure medications to adequately control blood pressure. Blood pressure can also be significantly improved in many people by means other than medications. Lifestyle changes such as reducing salt intake, exercising, losing weight if needed to reach "ideal" weight (see Chapter 15), and not smoking can all help reduce blood pressure.

Carotid, Aortic, and Peripheral Arterial Disease
Atherosclerosis, the disease that causes plaques and blockages to form in the coronary arteries, can also damage other arteries in the body. These include the

biggest artery of all, the aorta, and all the major arteries that come off the aorta.

The first three major arteries that come off the aortic after the coronary arteries are the brachiocephalic, left common carotid, and left subclavian arteries. All three arise, in that order, from the "aortic arch." This is the short part of the aorta shaped like an upside down "U" we talked about in the last chapter. The brachiocephalic artery quickly divides into the right subclavian artery and the right common carotid artery.

Each common carotid artery divides into an "external carotid" branch and an "internal carotid" branch. The two external carotid arteries supply blood to the face and neck. The two internal carotid arteries are the major arteries that supply blood to the brain.

The two subclavian arteries supply blood to the arms. Each subclavian artery has a branch called the vertebral artery. The right and left vertebral arteries run up the back of the neck and enter the bottom of the skull. There they join together to form the basilar artery, which supplies blood to the brainstem. Branches from the basilar artery also provide blood to parts of the brain in the back of the skull, such as the cerebellum.

Atherosclerotic blockages can form in any of these arteries. However, blockages in the "cerebral" arteries—the arteries that supply blood to the brain, especially the internal carotid arteries and their branches—are the most common and serious ones. If part of the brain doesn't get enough blood due to these blockages, the area of the body it controls won't work right. This can cause symptoms like loss of vision in one eye or part of both eyes, difficulty speaking, inability to move or feel an arm or leg, drooping of one side of the face, etc.

These blockages can cause problems with the brain not getting enough blood in two major ways. The degree of blockage in an internal carotid or other artery may become so severe that blood flow through the artery is significantly less than normal. However, people with only mild to moderate blockage in the arteries of their neck are also at increased risk of blocking off the blood supply to their brains. This is caused by a blood clot forming on an atherosclerotic plaque in a carotid or other cerebral artery. The clot then breaks off the plaque and travels "downstream" in the artery to the brain. Eventually the artery narrows down to a size too small for the blood clot to travel any farther. The blood clot then "plugs" the artery, interrupting blood flow to the part of the brain the artery supplies. Blood clots can also form directly on small arteries with blockages inside the brain itself.

A person is said to have a "transient ischemic attack" (TIA) if symptoms caused by the brain not getting enough blood go away within 24 hours. The problems with vision, speaking, etc. that occur with a TIA typically occur suddenly and usually last only minutes to hours. If symptoms persist for more than 24 hours, however, the person has had a stroke—also called a "cerebrovascular accident," or CVA. At least 15% of people who have a stroke had a TIA at some time before it. Each year about half a million people have a stroke for the first time. Another two hundred thousand people who've had a stroke before have a new one.

TIAs and strokes are usually caused by atherosclerotic blockages in the carotid artery and other cerebral arteries—"cerebrovascular disease." Treatment includes "blood thinning" medications such as aspirin, clopidogrel, and warfarin. As we'll discuss in Chapter 10, surgery and other procedures can also be used to treat severe blockage in the carotid arteries.

However, many other types of problems can also cause TIAs and strokes. The left atrium and left ventricle may contract so weakly that blood "pools" within them, forming a blood clot (thrombus). This blood clot can break off and travel through the aorta to one of the cerebral arteries. There the clot can block part of the blood supply to the brain.

A blood clot that forms in a vein can pass through a "patent foramen ovale" and cause a TIA or stroke. The foramen ovale is a small opening in the interatrial septum that separates the right atrium and the left atrium. The foramen ovale is normally open— "patent" —in a baby before it is born. In most people, the foramen ovale closes off within the first year after birth, so blood can't get directly from the right atrium to the left atrium. However, about 25% of people continue to have a patent foramen ovale later in life. In these people, a blood clot that forms in a vein can pass through the foramen ovale from the right atrium to the left atrium. From there the blood clot can travel through the left ventricle and aorta to reach the arteries of the brain and may cause a TIA or stroke.

Infected material ("vegetations") on the mitral or aortic valve can also break off, block the blood supply to the brain, and cause a TIA or stroke.

In about 15% of people, strokes are associated with bleeding within the brain itself. The causes for this bleeding include rupture of an artery within the brain and a head injury.

Severe atherosclerotic disease in a subclavian artery can cause pain and weakness in the arm it supplies with blood. A severe blockage in the part of the subclavian artery before the vertebral artery comes off it causes the "subclavian steal syndrome." Some of the blood in that vertebral artery actually flows "backwards" into the part of the subclavian artery beyond the blockage instead of going to the brain like it should. Raising or exercising the arm supplied by the diseased subclavian artery can make this problem worse. If the brain doesn't get enough blood, the person may experience dizziness, difficulty with balance, problems with vision, or even pass out.

As a person ages, the wall of the aorta may weaken. This can result in a widening ("aneurysm") of the aorta. An aortic aneurysm most commonly occurs in the abdomen (belly). An "abdominal aortic aneurysm" (AAA) may involve the aorta above or below where the arteries of the kidneys (the renal arteries) arise from the aorta. If the AAA involves the renal arteries, it can potentially causing problems with kidney function. The risk of having an AAA is higher in men than in women and increases with age. Most people with an AAA are more than 60 years old. Smokers are also significantly more likely to develop an AAA. Elderly male smokers have the greatest risk of developing an AAA.

An AAA may cause no symptoms. It may be detected only when a pulsating mass is found in the abdomen during a routine physical exam or may be seen on an imaging study such as an ultrasound test, CT scan, or magnetic resonance imaging (MRI). An AAA typically has a significant amount of atherosclerotic plaque within it. As they do in the cerebral arteries, atherosclerotic plaques inside the aneurysm can form blood clots on them. Cholesterol crystals can also form on these plaques. These blood clots and crystals can break off and interrupt the blood supply to the legs. This can cause a bluish-purple discoloration of the feet and toes—"blue toe syndrome."

The most serious danger with an AAA is that it can rupture and cause life-threatening bleeding. A person may develop sudden pain, often described as a "tearing" pain in the middle of the lower part of the back. This can cause the person to become lightheaded and pass out due to bleeding around the aneurysm. The chance that an AAA will rupture increases significantly when the AAA becomes wider than a little over two inches in diameter. Albert Einstein died of a ruptured AAA. As we'll discuss in Chapter 10, surgery can be done to treat an aortic aneurysm before it ruptures.

Aortic aneurysms also occur in the part of the aorta within the chest—a "thoracic" aortic aneurysm. Thoracic aortic aneurysms are less common than AAAs. Like an AAA, a thoracic aortic aneurysm is caused by the aorta's wall becoming weak. In the elderly this is usually caused by "arteriosclerosis"— thickening and hardening of an artery's walls—and "cystic medial degeneration." Thoracic aortic aneurysms usually do not produce symptoms. However, they may cause pain in the chest or back and can also rupture. Aneurysms in the first or "ascending" part of the aorta can cause the aortic valve to leak.

The inner lining of the aorta can tear due to high blood pressure or an abnormality in the wall of the aorta. This "aortic dissection" causes blood to be pumped with each heartbeat into an abnormal space ("false lumen") within the wall of the aorta itself. This causes more tearing within the aorta's wall and can lead to rupture of the aorta. Aortic dissection most commonly occurs within the ascending aorta, but it can occur anywhere within the aorta. An aortic dissection typically causes severe, "tearing" pain. A dissection involving the first two parts of the aorta, the ascending aorta and aortic arch, can cause pain in the chest and neck. A dissection in the descending aorta, the part beyond the aortic arch, can cause pain in the back.

Dissection of the ascending aorta at the level of the aortic valve can even block off the openings to the coronary arteries, causing a heart attack. If the dissection involves the aortic arch and blocks off the openings of the arteries supplying blood to the brain, it can cause symptoms of a stroke. A new dissection of the ascending aorta or aortic arch needs emergency treatment. This type of dissection requires surgery to repair or replace the part of the aorta where the dissection started. A new dissection of the "descending" aorta—the part beyond the arch—may require surgery. Sometimes, however, a dissection of the descending aorta can be successfully treated with medication alone. The medications used to treat a new aortic dissection slow the heart rate and lower blood pressure. This reduces the "shearing" effects of the blood pumped out with each beat on the aorta.

Atherosclerotic plaques commonly occur in thoracic aortic aneurysms, particularly in older people. Thoracic aortic aneurysms can also be caused by inflammation or infection. For example, people with untreated syphilis can develop a thoracic aortic aneurysm many years after they became infected. Surgery to repair or replace the aneurysm to prevent rupture is typically done when the thoracic aneurysm is about two and one half inches in diameter.

People with a genetic disorder called Marfan's syndrome have a particularly high risk of developing an ascending aortic aneurysm. They have a defect in the elastic tissue in their bodies that is associated with multiple abnormalities. These include eye problems; unusually long fingers, arms and legs; and joints that bend more than usual. This genetic defect also weakens the walls of the aorta and can cause an ascending aortic aneurysm to develop even in people as young as their teens and twenties. The ascending aortic aneurysms seen in people with Marfan's syndrome can eventually rupture or dissect. Surgery to replace the diseased part of the aorta in people with Marfan's syndrome is typically done when the aneurysm is about two inches in width.

"Peripheral arterial disease" refers to atherosclerotic blockages that develop in the arteries of the legs and, much less commonly, the arms. It is estimated that about eight to ten million Americans have peripheral arterial disease. The main symptom associated with this problem is "claudication"—either pain or a feeling of fatigue or aching within the part of the body that's not getting enough blood. Moderate blockage in the arteries of the legs causes "intermittent" claudication— discomfort that occurs with exertion, like walking, and is relieved by rest. Blockages in arteries farther down in the leg typically cause pain in the calves, while those higher up in the leg cause pain in the hip, thigh, and buttocks. If there are significant blockages in the arteries that supply blood to the penis and other genitals, this can cause sexual dysfunction, such as inability to achieve or maintain an erection.

Severe blockages in the arteries of the legs can cause claudication even when a person isn't walking. The toes and feet may develop ulcers that don't heal and even turn black and die from lack of blood. Other potential signs and symptoms of peripheral arterial disease include: numbness or weakness of the legs; cold feet or legs; reddish or bluish discoloration of the feet (especially when sitting or standing); and hair loss on the feet and legs.

A variety of medications are now used to treat peripheral arterial disease. These include: "blood thinning" medications such as aspirin, clopidogrel, or warfarin; cholesterol-lowering medications; and other medicines such as cilostazol (Pletal), pentoxifylline, or calcium antagonists. As we'll discuss in Chapter 10, surgery and other procedures are also effective for treating peripheral arterial disease. It's particularly important that a person with peripheral arterial disease avoid smoking. Nicotine and other harmful substances in tobacco make arteries "clamp down" and further reduce blood and oxygen to the legs and other parts of the body supplied by arteries with blockages.

The risk factors for developing carotid artery disease, aortic disease, and peripheral arterial disease are similar to those for CAD. These risk factors include smoking, high blood pressure, high cholesterol, and diabetes. Not surprisingly, a person with an AAA or peripheral arterial disease is also very likely to have CAD, whether he or she knows it or not. While people with carotid artery disease also have an increased risk of having CAD, this risk is lower than in people with peripheral arterial disease.

CAD, heart failure, hypertension, and diseases of the body's arteries are the most serious and common problems affecting the heart and blood vessels. In the next chapter, we'll discuss what else can go wrong with the heart and blood vessels.

Chapter 5 Summary
- ♥ Coronary artery disease is caused by atherosclerosis and is the leading cause of death in adult Americans.

- ♥ Coronary artery blockages cause myocardial ischemia, the condition in which the heart muscle does not get enough blood and oxygen.

- ♥ Prolonged myocardial ischemia may lead to a heart attack.

- ♥ The overall risk of having a heart attack during sex is very small.

- ♥ Smoking, high blood pressure, diabetes, and high cholesterol increase a person's risk of developing coronary artery disease, heart failure, aortic disease, and blockages in arteries to the brain and the rest of the body.

Chapter 6: From Valves to Veins
Other Major Causes of Heart Problems

Chapter Preview
Diseases of the Heart Valves
    Aortic valve disease
    Mitral valve disease
    Rheumatic fever
Infective Endocarditis
    Infection of heart valves
    Causes and risk factors
    Treatment and prevention
Heart Tumors
    Benign tumors (myxoma)
    Malignant tumors
Pericardial Disease
    Pericarditis
    Pericardial fluid collection (effusion)
Congenital Heart Disease
    Simple and complicated
Arrhythmias
    Bradyarrythmias (slow heart rhythms)
    Premature ("skipped") heart beats
    Atrial fibrillation and atrial flutter
    Other tachyarrhythmias (fast heart rhythms)
Deep Vein Thrombosis and Pulmonary Embolism
    Causes of blood clots in veins
    Blood clots in the lungs (pulmonary embolism)

IN THE LAST chapter we concentrated mainly on problems involving the arteries of the heart and the rest of the body. In this chapter we'll focus on problems involving other structures of the heart.

Diseases of the Heart Valves

Diseases involving the heart valves can occur in both young and old people. The diseases are far more likely to involve the aortic and mitral valves than the tricuspid or pulmonic valves. The aortic and mitral valves can have problems with abnormal narrowing—"stenosis"—or leaking—"regurgitation" or "insufficiency."

Aortic stenosis is mainly a disease of older people. It may occur partly due to "wear and tear" on the valve as a person ages. Aortic stenosis can also be due to degeneration and inflammation of the valve associated with the same risk factors as CAD, including hypertension, high cholesterol, etc. As the valve is damaged the body deposits hard, rock-like calcium on it, blocking its opening. If the opening of the aortic valve becomes too narrow, a person may develop heart failure, pass out, have angina—and may even die suddenly.

In a small percentage of people with aortic stenosis, the aortic valve was abnormal at birth. A baby with this abnormality usually has only mild to moderate aortic stenosis. However, the aortic stenosis may be so severe that it is life-threatening. About 1% of people are born with a "bicuspid" aortic valve—a valve that has only two leaflets instead of the normal three leaflets. A bicuspid aortic valve usually starts out as having no significant narrowing. However, a bicuspid aortic valve has a greater chance of becoming stenotic and of doing so at an earlier age (on average, about a decade or two sooner) than someone who starts out with a normal aortic valve.

Aortic regurgitation can occur from infection or inflammation of the valve, disease (especially widening) of the part of the aorta just above the valve, traumatic injury (like a serious car accident) or, uncommonly, rheumatoid arthritis and other diseases that primarily affect other parts of the body. With each heartbeat, some of the blood the left ventricle pumps out into the aorta comes back into the ventricle again through the leaking aortic valve. Over time the left ventricle enlarges and weakens due to the excess strain of having to pump out a good portion of the blood it just sent out with one heartbeat all over again with the next one. People with significant aortic regurgitation can develop shortness of breath, heart failure, fatigue, palpitations and, in severe cases, angina. However, they may not develop any symptoms at all until the left ventricle is significantly enlarged and weakened.

Similar problems occur in people with mitral regurgitation. Here, part of the blood the left ventricle tries to pump out only into the aorta leaks back through the mitral valve into the left atrium. This blood returns to the left ventricle during diastole when the mitral valve opens. Mitral regurgitation has many causes. It can be due to tearing or injury to part of the valve such as can occur with a heart attack. If the left ventricle enlarges for any reason the mitral valve can be an "innocent bystander," stretched apart enough that its two leaflets can't close properly.

One or both of the mitral valve leaflets can "prolapse." This means the leaflet buckles back into the left atrium when the left ventricle is contracting. This can allow blood to leak back through the mitral valve and cause mitral regurgitation. Mitral valve prolapse can be seen in young people, especially young women. It is usually benign when present in young people, with most of them having mild or no regurgitation. However, mitral valve prolapse in older people is typically due to degeneration of the valve and is more likely to cause significant mitral regurgitation and other problems.

Less common causes of mitral regurgitation include damage to the valve from infection, trauma, diseases that affect the joints like rheumatoid arthritis and systemic lupus erythematosus, and a disease we discussed in the last chapter, hypertrophic obstructive cardiomyopathy.

The symptoms and problems associated with mitral regurgitation are similar to those seen with aortic regurgitation. Mitral regurgitation can cause shortness of breath and other symptoms of heart failure and may increase the risk of having abnormal heart rhythms. The left ventricle responds in a manner similar to how it responds to severe aortic regurgitation. Initially the left ventricle contracts more forcefully. However, as it begins to fail the left ventricle contracts less forcefully and increases in size.

Mitral stenosis, or narrowing of the mitral valve, is by far most commonly caused by a problem that can affect all four heart valves and the heart muscle itself—rheumatic fever. Heart disease due to rheumatic fever is much less common in the United States than it was several generations ago. However, worldwide it continues to be the most common cause of acquired heart disease in children and young adults. The risk of having rheumatic fever is highest in children ages 6 to 15. Rheumatic fever occurs about three weeks after an episode of streptococcus A pharyngitis—"strep throat." However, only a few percent of people having this infection will develop rheumatic fever. Treatment with antibiotics such as penicillin virtually eliminates the chance that rheumatic fever will occur.

However, if a person has had an episode of rheumatic fever before, the chance of having it after another bout of strep throat is much higher—about 50%. People who have had rheumatic fever require long-term use of penicillin, with injections typically given every month until age 21, to prevent this disease from occurring again. If the heart was damaged significantly during a person's previous bout with rheumatic fever, penicillin injections may need to be given for the rest of the person's life.

Most symptoms of rheumatic fever, like joint pains, fever, rash, and skin nodules (lumps) last no more than several weeks and don't cause any long-term damage. However, this disease can damage the heart with a "one-two" punch. During the episode of rheumatic fever itself the heart muscle, heart valves, and tissue surrounding the heart (pericardium) can all become inflamed. Damage to the heart muscle is only occasionally severe enough to cause congestive heart failure and only rarely results in death. Damaged heart muscle usually recovers after rheumatic fever resolves. Inflammation of the heart valves caused by rheumatic fever can result in mitral regurgitation and aortic regurgitation. However, the degree of valve regurgitation is usually only mild.

This inflammation of the heart and its valves typically improves after a few weeks. However, a significant minority of people will develop worse heart valve problems years later. Scar tissue slowly forms on these damaged valves over the following years. As little as a decade after an episode of rheumatic fever the mitral valve may become significantly narrowed, limiting the flow of blood from the left atrium to the left ventricle.

If mitral stenosis is severe enough it can produce disabling shortness of breath, heart failure due to not enough blood getting through the narrowed mitral valve, chest pain, coughing up blood, abnormal heart rhythms like atrial fibrillation (see below), and pulmonary hypertension. The risk of blood clots forming in the left atrium is significant, especially if atrial fibrillation is present. These blood clots can break off and travel out of the heart, blocking off the blood supply to the brain and causing a stroke, or damaging other organs in the same way.

While mitral stenosis is the most common long-term heart problem associated with rheumatic fever, it can also cause various combinations of mitral regurgitation, aortic regurgitation, and aortic stenosis—even in the same person. Rheumatic fever can also cause stenosis and regurgitation of the tricuspid and pulmonic valves. However, rheumatic fever is much less likely to significantly damage these two right-sided heart valves than it is to damage the aortic and mitral valves.

Infective Endocarditis
Another kind of heart valve problem that can affect any of the four valves is infective endocarditis. This is an infection of one or more of the heart valves. As with rheumatic fever, the mitral valve and the aortic valve are much more likely to be involved than the tricuspid or pulmonic valves. Infective endocarditis can occur on normal heart valves. However, it is more likely to occur if the valve is already abnormal or damaged, especially if it is an artificial heart valve from prior valve replacement surgery.

Bacteria cause most cases of infective endocarditis, although fungi and other microorganisms can do it too. Normal heart valves tend to be attacked by more aggressive bacteria, like *Staphylococcus aureus*, while abnormal or artificial valves are more likely to be infected by somewhat less virulent ones, such as streptococci. The infected valve can be damaged directly by the organism, possibly causing severe regurgitation of the valve. Abnormal masses (vegetations) can also form on the valve leaflets. These vegetations can grow large enough to partially block off the valve. Parts of these vegetations can even shed off and, as with the runaway blood clots we've discussed before, cause stroke or damage other organs. An abscess—a collection of pus—can also form, especially around the aortic valve, where it can even interfere with the electrical conducting system of the heart.

While most cases of endocarditis involve abnormal valves, it may also occur without any obvious cause. The risk of developing endocarditis is increased in people with illnesses that have reduced their resistance to infection, or who have procedures (like extensive dental work, or surgery on organs like the intestines or bladder) that cause more bacteria to be temporarily released into the bloodstream. Intravenous drug abusers have an increased risk of developing endocarditis due to their use of contaminated needles and injecting other infectious material into their veins. They are more likely to have endocarditis involving the tricuspid and pulmonic valves than other people with endocarditis.

Fever is the most common symptom associated with endocarditis. Depending on which heart valve(s) are involved and how severe the infection is, a person with endocarditis may also have shortness of breath, sweating, loss of appetite, confusion, and evidence of a stroke or damage to other organs. Endocarditis is always fatal if it is not treated. Treatment with appropriate antibiotics and, in some cases, replacement of the infected valve significantly improves the chances of survival. The particular antibiotics and antifungal agents used to treat endocarditis are based on which microorganism caused the infection. The microorganism is identified by obtaining blood samples and culturing them or, occasionally, by culturing infected tissue. Antibiotics are typically given for about four to six weeks.

As stated above, people with abnormal heart valves and some other kinds of heart problems have a greater risk of developing infective endocarditis after certain procedures and surgery. These include some types of dental work and operations on the stomach, gallbladder, prostate gland, and bladder. The risk of getting infective endocarditis is increased due to these procedures causing a greater number of bacteria to be briefly released into the bloodstream. Taking certain antibiotics shortly before and, in some cases, a short time after these procedures is recommended to reduce the risk of endocarditis in these people.

Heart Tumors
It's uncommon for tumors or cancer to involve the heart. A cancer in the heart is usually a "metastasis" —a part of a cancer that originated in some other part of the body and spread to the heart. When a tumor does develop in the heart it is usually "benign" and not a cancer. Tumors inside the heart can cause problems by restricting blood flow within the heart. Part of the tumor may also "shed" off it and block the blood supply to part of the body.

In adults, the most common tumor that begins in the heart is a myxoma. A myxoma is a benign tumor that can be seen even in young adults. The myxoma is usually attached to the interatrial septum and located in the left atrium. However, this tumor can occur in the other heart chambers too. Myxomas can grow quite large, partially blocking off the opening of the mitral valve and mimicking mitral stenosis. Part of the myxoma can also break off and cause a stroke. A person with a myxoma needs to have an operation to remove it. However, sometimes myxomas grow back after surgery.

Rhabdomyomas are rare, benign tumors involving the walls of the left ventricle or right ventricle. A rhabdomyoma is more likely to occur in a child than in an adult.

When a true cancer like an angiosarcoma or rhabdomyosarcoma does develop in the heart, treatment with surgery can be difficult. These rare tumors can spread to other parts of the body. Chemotherapy or radiation therapy may be effective in some cases.

Pericardial Disease

The pericardium, the tissue that surrounds the heart like a bag, can also develop problems. "Pericarditis" occurs when the pericardium become inflamed, usually due to a viral infection. People with pericarditis may have shortness of breath, fever, or sharp chest pains. Problems with the heart itself, the pericardium, and sometimes other parts of the body (such as kidney failure or cancer) can cause fluid to accumulate between the pericardium and the heart—a "pericardial effusion." If the pericardial effusion grows too rapidly or is too large, it can even interfere with the heart's function—"pericardial tamponade." The fluid may need to be drained with a needle and syringe or by having a surgeon open up the pericardium.

"Constrictive pericarditis" occurs when the pericardium become scarred and thickened due to an earlier episode of inflammation and injury. This can be caused by previous infections, like viral pericarditis or tuberculosis; prior radiation to the chest, such as for treatment of a cancer; old heart surgery; or a heart attack. Calcium may be deposited in the pericardium, making it hard and rock-like. This tight pericardium constricts the heart, preventing its chambers from filling with blood the way they should. Pressures increase in all four of the heart chambers. A person may experience shortness of breath, fatigue, lightheadedness, chest pain, and swelling in the belly and legs. Surgery may be needed to "strip" the pericardium away from the heart.

Congenital Heart Disease
There are a large number of "congenital" heart defects —abnormalities in the heart, its valves, or the blood vessels connected to it that are present from birth. We'll discuss them in detail in later chapters. For now, we'll just say that some are relatively "simple" defects. For example, an atrial septal defect is an abnormal opening in the interatrial septum, the tissue separating the right atrium and left atrium. This causes abnormal blood flow from the left atrium to the right atrium. A small atrial septal defect may not cause any symptoms and might not even be discovered until adulthood. A ventricular septal defect is an abnormal opening in the interventricular septum, the tissue that separates the left ventricle from the right ventricle. Blood travels through the ventricular septal defect from the left ventricle to the right ventricle. A small ventricular septal defect might close by itself during childhood.

Other congenital heart defects are more complicated. They require surgery to at least partially correct the abnormalities in the heart and its major blood vessels. Some congenital heart defects are so severe a baby or child may die without surgery. Fortunately, many procedures and operations are now available to help treat even severe congenital heart defects.

Arrhythmias

The last major category of heart problems we'll discuss here is abnormal heart rhythms—"arrhythmias." Arrhythmias can be roughly grouped into three major categories—those that cause abnormally slow, normal, and fast heart rates. Arrhythmias are also classified according to where they originate. A "supraventricular" arrhythmia begins within an atrium or the AV node. As the name implies, a "ventricular" arrhythmia begins within a ventricle.

Bradyarrhythmias—abnormally slow heart rates—can be due to problems anywhere within the electrical system of the heart. The sinus node, where electrical impulses normally originate, may send fewer impulses than it should down through the rest of the electrical system—"sinus node dysfunction." This can happen if the sinus node doesn't get enough blood or if it is injured, such as during a heart attack. Certain medications and diseases, like hypothyroidism (low thyroid function), can also suppress the sinus node. They can cause "sinus bradycardia," a heart rhythm controlled by the sinus node but with a heart rate less than 60 beats per minute.

Farther down in the heart's electrical system, the AV node can also be affected by these same kinds of problems. In this case, the sinus node is sending the right number of electrical impulses, but not all of these impulses are getting through the AV node to the ventricles. The degree of "AV block" may vary from just the rare electrical impulse that doesn't get through, to all of these electrical impulses getting blocked—"complete heart block." In the latter case, if the person is to stay alive the AV node itself has to generate electrical impulses that can travel on down to the ventricles. The AV node normally produces these impulses at the rate of 40 to 60 beats per minute. This heart rate is enough to sustain life, but is it is low enough for a person to possibly have shortness of breath or other symptoms.

Sometimes the abnormal AV node doesn't produce enough impulses to give an adequate heart rate. At other times, the sinus node and AV node may be working right, but the level of blocked impulses is even farther down the heart's electrical system, in the ventricles. In either case, the ventricles become the "last hope" for the person to generate electrical impulses fast enough to sustain life. Unfortunately, the ventricles usually generate electrical impulses on their own at a rate of only about 20 to 30 beats per minute. A heart rate this slow is unlikely to supply an adequate amount of blood to the rest of the body, especially the brain. Sometimes the ventricles produce virtually no electrical impulses at all. Then the heart goes into "asystole," with no electrical activity or heartbeat. In either case, unless something is done very quickly the person is not long for this world.

The most common arrhythmias that occur when the heart rate is normal (60 to 100 beats per minute) are premature atrial contractions (PACs) and premature ventricular contractions (PVCs). These are beats that originate, not in the sinus node, but either within an atrium (PACs) or a ventricle (PVCs). PACs and PVCs typically occur when a person is in a normal, sinus rhythm. However, they occur early (hence the "premature" part of the name), before the next sinus beat is due. A person may feel them as an "extra" or "skipped" beat.

PACs and PVCs can occur one at a time or in pairs (couplets). They can also occur randomly or in a fairly regular pattern. PACs and PVCs occur commonly in people with significant heart problems such as CAD or cardiomyopathy. However, many people with PACs and PVCs don't have any other heart problem. In these otherwise normal people, PACs and PVCs may cause annoying palpitations but aren't associated with anything more serious. Low doses of certain medications such as beta-blockers, diltiazem, or verapamil can be used to suppress PACs and PVCs if they do cause significant palpitations.

Drinking alcohol or beverages containing caffeine such as coffee, tea, or soda can cause or worsen PACs and PVCs. So can taking certain medications like pseudoephedrine, a medicine used to treat a runny nose. PACs and PVCs can also be caused by medical problems not due to the heart itself, such as a low level of potassium in the blood or abnormally high thyroid function (hyperthyroidism).

Accelerated junctional rhythm and accelerated idioventricular rhythm are arrhythmias that can produce heart rates in the normal range. In accelerated junctional rhythm, increased irritability of the AV node due to reduced blood supply or other causes, such as certain medications, can make the AV node generate electrical impulses in the "normal" range of 60 to 100 beats per minute. This rate can be faster than the rate the sinus node is producing electrical impulses. In that case, accelerated junctional rhythm becomes the dominant heart rhythm instead of sinus rhythm. Accelerated idioventricular rhythm has similar characteristics and causes, except electrical impulses originate in one of the ventricles instead of the AV node.

The third category of arrhythmias is "tachyarrhythmias." These are arrhythmias that cause a fast heart rate of more than 100 beats per minute. Tachyarrhythmias can be subdivided into those that originate in an atrium or the AV node ("supraventricular tachyarrhythmias") and those generated in a ventricle ("ventricular tachyarrhythmias"). The major types of supraventricular tachyarrhythmias are atrial flutter, atrial fibrillation, and paroxysmal supraventricular tachycardia. Ventricular tachyarrhythmias include two types we discussed in Chapter 5, ventricular tachycardia and ventricular fibrillation. This category also includes several specific types of ventricular tachycardia—ventricular flutter, polymorphous ventricular tachycardia, and torsades de pointes.

Atrial fibrillation is the most common of these arrhythmias. It becomes more common as a person gets older. Atrial fibrillation is present in at least 5% of people who are at least 70 years old. The risk of developing atrial fibrillation is higher in people with significant heart disease, especially those with a weakened left ventricle or mitral stenosis. Atrial fibrillation can also be caused by problems in parts of the body besides the heart, like hyperthyroidism caused by an overactive thyroid gland. The same substances and medications we described earlier that cause PACs can also produce atrial fibrillation. This arrhythmia can even occur in young people with no other obvious heart problems—"lone fibrillators."

With atrial fibrillation, too many electrical impulses (about 500 or more) are generated within the atria for them to contract. Instead of pumping blood, the atria just "quiver." This is similar to what happens with ventricular fibrillation. However, while ventricular fibrillation can make a person die within a matter of minutes, atrial fibrillation is only rarely life-threatening. While the ventricles are the primary pumps for the heart and need to move blood so a person can live, the atria aren't absolutely necessary for this.

The atria only contract near the end of diastole (the so-called "atrial kick"), usually contributing about 20% of the total amount of blood the ventricles are going to pump out with the next heartbeat. When this 20% contribution is lost with atrial fibrillation, people generally either don't feel a difference or only feel more easily fatigued. There are exceptions, however. People with certain heart problems, like mitral stenosis or hypertrophic obstructive cardiomyopathy, are likely to develop significant symptoms with atrial fibrillation. These people need their left atrium to contract to force more blood into the left ventricle.

How much a person is affected by atrial fibrillation also depends on what their heart rate is with this arrhythmia. With atrial fibrillation, the atria generate many hundreds of impulses per minute and send them on to the AV node. However, the AV node can't conduct all of these impulses to the ventricles. This is a good thing, since a person couldn't live for long if their ventricles were contracting several hundred times per minute.

The number of impulses the AV node is able to conduct varies a great deal. Unless medications are used to block the AV node, the number of electrical impulses that get through to the ventricles typically is somewhere from 100 to 170 every minute. This produces an abnormally fast and irregular heart rate. The heart rate may be fast enough to give a person chest pain, shortness of breath, or other symptoms. In older individuals, the AV node may conduct fewer impulses.

They may have a heart rate that is within the normal range of 60 to 100 beats per minute, or even slower.

Another major problem with atrial fibrillation is that, since the atria aren't contracting and pumping blood, this blood can pool inside them. This can make blood clots form in the atria. A blood clot in the left atrium can break off and travel through the mitral valve and left ventricle into the aorta. From there the blood clot can block one of the arteries that supply blood to the brain and cause a stroke. The risk of stroke with atrial fibrillation is low in an otherwise healthy person less than 60 years old. The risk of stroke is higher in people who are at least 60 years old, particularly those 75 years old or older. This risk is also higher in people with diabetes, hypertension, CAD, and a prior stroke. The risk of stroke with atrial fibrillation is particularly great when left ventricular systolic function is at least mildly lower than normal or if a person has mitral stenosis.

Similar problems occur in people with atrial flutter. In this rhythm, the atria generate abnormal impulses at a rate of about 250 to 350 per minute. Usually, only half or fewer of these impulses get through the AV node to the ventricles. The heart rate can be fast or even normal, depending on how many of these impulses get through. As with atrial fibrillation, the atria don't contract efficiently with atrial flutter. People with atrial flutter have an increased risk of blood clots forming in the atria and of having a stroke.

Both atrial fibrillation and atrial flutter may go away without any treatment. If either arrhythmia persists, certain medications may help to make the heart go back into normal rhythm. Atrial fibrillation and atrial flutter can also be treated with "electrical cardioversion." In this procedure the person first receives intravenous medications to reduce discomfort and make the individual go to sleep. The heart is then shocked through two patches placed on the chest and connected to an external cardioverter-defibrillator. Alternatively, one patch is placed on the left side of the chest over the heart and the other patch directly behind it on the left side of the back.

Paroxysmal supraventricular tachycardia (PSVT) comes in several varieties. This arrhythmia typically involves an electrical impulse that "gets lost" within the AV node due to abnormal conduction, generating a large number of additional, rapid electrical impulses. PSVT may also involve an abnormal area of tissue (bypass tract) that a small percentage of people have. The bypass tract causes abnormal conduction of electrical impulses between a ventricle and an atrium.

PSVT typically causes a heart rate between 150 and 250 beats per minute. Unlike atrial fibrillation or flutter, it is most commonly seen for the first time in younger adults. PSVT may stop spontaneously or go away with certain maneuvers, like straining or gagging. If needed, medications can be used or the heart can be shocked to stop the arrhythmia and restore normal rhythm.

Ventricular tachycardia is an abnormal heart rhythm that originates in a ventricle. It is defined as at least three ventricular beats in a row at a rate of at least 110 beats per minute. Ventricular tachycardia is "nonsustained" if it lasts continuously for less than thirty seconds and "sustained" if it lasts longer. It is usually "monomorphic." This means the abnormal complexes—the tracings seen on an electrocardiogram (EKG), a test that records the heart's electrical activity—look about the same.

Ventricular flutter is a form of monomorphic ventricular tachycardia with a particular monotonous pattern of complexes. It typically occurs at a rate of about 300 beats per minute. Ventricular flutter is life-threatening due to its fast rate.

"Polymorphous" ventricular tachycardia differs from the typical monomorphic variety in that it shows different sizes and shapes of ventricular complexes on an EKG. Torsades de pointes is a specific type of polymorphous ventricular tachycardia. It is characterized by a distinctive "twisting" pattern of ventricular complexes. Torsades de pointes usually occurs at a rate of about 200 to 250 beats per minute. Its significance is that it occurs in specific situations, such as abnormally slow heart rates, a low level of minerals like potassium in the blood, and with use of certain medications. Torsades de pointes is also associated with a particular abnormality on the EKG, a "long Q-T interval." It is also treated somewhat differently than other types of ventricular tachycardia. Certain medications that can suppress other types of ventricular tachycardia may actually make torsades de pointes worse. Like other types of ventricular tachycardia, a shock to the chest using a cardioverter-defibrillator can end torsades de pointes and restore normal rhythm.

Deep Vein Thrombosis and Pulmonary Embolism
Blood clots in the veins of the legs and, less commonly, other parts of the body can also cause indirect problems for the heart. These blood clots are more likely to form when a person hasn't been moving for a while. This can happen when someone has been sitting in a car or airplane for many hours during a trip or has been ill enough to be bedridden, such as after surgery or if the person is in a nursing home. Other causes of

these blood clots include use of birth control pills, estrogen replacement therapy in postmenopausal women, pregnancy, injury (which can be major or minor, and can include broken bones), and cancer.

If a "deep vein thrombosis"—the technical name for a blood clot in one of these veins—stays in the leg, it can cause pain, swelling, redness, and tenderness there. However, deep vein thrombosis may not cause any symptoms at all. The blood clot may resolve by itself over time. However, usually the best treatment for a deep vein thrombosis that occurs above the level of the knee is to use medications that thin the blood.

Sometimes a blood clot breaks off from its place in a vein in the leg or other part of the body. The blood clot travels with the rest of the blood in the veins to the right side of the heart. From there the blood clot passes into the arteries in the lungs (pulmonary arteries). Eventually the blood clot stops when it gets to a part of a pulmonary artery that's too small to let it move any farther. This is called "pulmonary embolism." The blood clot keeps blood from reaching part of the lung. The affected section of the lung is prevented from doing its usual job of exchanging carbon dioxide for oxygen in the blood. Pulmonary embolism can also put strain on the right ventricle, which has to pump against an increased pressure caused by the blood clot "plugging" part of the pulmonary arteries.

Pulmonary embolism can make a person short of breath and breathe faster. This is because not as much oxygen is getting into the blood. Pulmonary embolism can also cause sharp chest pains and a fast heart rate. Sometimes it makes a person cough up blood and may damage part of the lung. With a large pulmonary embolism, one or more blood clots block off so much of the pulmonary arteries that not enough blood gets through to the left side of the heart. This can cause a person's blood pressure to fall to a dangerous level. The individual may feel lightheaded, pass out, or even die. Blood thinners are used to treat pulmonary embolism. In the most severe cases, surgery can be done to remove blood clots from the pulmonary arteries.

As we've seen in this chapter, the heart and blood vessels form a complex system that, while very reliable, can malfunction. In later chapters we'll discuss how broken hearts can be mended.

Chapter 6 Summary

- ♥ Diseases of the heart valves can cause heart failure and other problems.

- ♥ In general, it is uncommon for tumors or cancer to involve the heart.

- ♥ Inflammation, infection, or injury can lead to disease of the pericardium, the thin sac-like tissue that surround the heart.

- ♥ Abnormal heart rhythms (arrhythmias) can cause the heart rate to be too slow, too fast, or may produce "skipped" beats.

- ♥ Birth control pills are one potential cause of blood clots in the legs and lungs.

Chapter 7: Heart Attack!
Recognizing and Treating a Heart Attack

Chapter Preview:
Introduction
Initial Treatment of a Heart Attack
    Initial tests
    "MONA" medications
"Blood Thinners" for Heart Attacks
    Heparin
    Clopidogrel
Beta-Blockers and Other Medications
    Effects of beta-blockers
    Angiotensin-converting enzyme (ACE) inhibitors
    Angiotensin receptor blockers (ARBs)
Arrhythmias and Heart Attacks
    Ventricular fibrillation and ventricular tachycardia
    Automatic external defibrillator
    External transthoracic pacemaker
    Temporary transvenous pacemaker
    Antiarrhythmic medications
Evaluation of Chest Pain
    Clinical assessment
    Cardiac enzymes
    Electrocardiogram (EKG)
Inside the Intensive Care Unit
    Medications
    Swan-Ganz catheter
    Intra-aortic balloon pump
Thrombolytic Treatment and Coronary Angiography
    Thrombolytic medications
    Coronary angiography

THE WAYS HEART problems are diagnosed and treated have advanced dramatically over the past few decades, particularly since the late 1960s. To illustrate this, let's review what the state of the art was for treating a patient with a myocardial infarction—more commonly called a heart attack or "coronary"—back in 1965. That was one year after the Surgeon General released the first major report on the hazards of smoking.

Let's make our hypothetical patient a 50-year-old man, a smoker (like 52% of American men were that year), overweight (information about the full benefits of exercise and watching cholesterol wasn't available yet), and with high blood pressure. If he had ventricular fibrillation with his heart attack as he was strolling down a sidewalk, he would be out of luck. Techniques for performing cardiopulmonary resuscitation (CPR) were still in their infancy, and the training of lay people to do it had just begun. Defibrillators to shock his heart back into a normal rhythm were available in hospitals. However, these early defibrillators were too large and bulky to carry on ambulances. By the time our poor patient reached the emergency room (ER), the odds are very high he would just be pronounced dead from "the big one."

Now let's be more optimistic and have our patient with a heart attack arrive at the hospital alive. A doctor or nurse would obtain a history and do a physical examination on him. Our patient would also have an electrocardiogram (EKG), a test that measures the electrical activity of the heart, and a chest X-ray done. Treatment could include putting a nitroglycerin tablet under his tongue or breaking a glass capsule of amyl nitrate under his nose and letting him inhale the fumes. The patient would then typically be admitted to the hospital and placed in an oxygen tent. He would not be placed in a special intensive care unit for heart patients—a coronary care unit or "CCU," equipped with heart monitors and other special equipment—for the simple reason these units weren't fully developed until the late 1960s. Then he'd be kept at bed rest for weeks or months afterward—if he survived that long!

And that's it. Except for the EKG, chest X-ray, and nitroglycerin tablet, none of the standard tests and treatments we use today were either routinely done or even available back then.

Initial Treatment of a Heart Attack
Let's compare this to how the same patient would be treated now. First, it's less likely that he would be a smoker. While over half of American men smoked in 1965, less than 25% do now. Even if our patient continues to smoke, at least he's been advised by the Surgeon General's warning on every pack of cigarettes and by his own doctor of the hazards of smoking. His physician would also have obtained blood tests to check for diabetes, high cholesterol, and other factors that would put the patient at increased risk for a heart attack. If he had told his doctor he was having chest pains before he actually had the heart attack, a number of tests could have been done to see whether these pains might be due to coronary artery disease (CAD) or to another heart problem. We'll describe these other tests in the next chapter. Hopefully, by following his doctor's advice and doing everything he could to reduce his risk, the chances of him having a heart attack would have been significantly reduced.

On the other hand, if our patient did have a heart attack and collapsed in the street, hopefully someone nearby would start CPR and another bystander would call 911. An emergency vehicle with trained paramedics, equipped with a small portable defibrillator and a whole case full of medications, should arrive quickly to stabilize him for transfer to a hospital. The paramedics will start an intravenous (IV) line to give him any needed medications and start him on oxygen.

When our patient arrives at the ER, as in 1965, a chest X-ray and an EKG would still be done, with the latter having a higher priority. The EKG is useful for detecting abnormalities in the heart's rhythm and problems with the electrical conduction system of the heart. It can also help tell whether a person has had an old heart attack or is having one right now. Most people with heart attacks will have no changes on the EKG or changes that may or may not indicate a heart attack. Over a third, however, do have abnormalities on the EKG—"ST-elevation myocardial infarction"— that indicate there is an urgent need for certain medications and procedures we'll discuss later.

The basic treatment used if a person is found to have a heart attack or is suspected of having one includes "MONA" medications. The "M" stands for morphine. It is given through an IV line to relieve pain. Morphine can help reduce the amount of work the heart has to do by decreasing the amount of venous blood returning to it. While it doesn't treat the underlying problem, it can help make the patient more comfortable until more definitive treatment can be given.

"O" stands for oxygen. The oxygen can be delivered through tubes placed in the nose, by mask or, in someone who has stopped breathing or is very short of breath, by a tube placed down the throat, such as an endotracheal tube. As we discussed in Chapter 5, a heart attack occurs when an area of the heart doesn't get enough blood and oxygen. Increasing the amount of oxygen a person breathes may, to some degree, help the heart get more of the oxygen it needs.

"N" stands for nitroglycerin. This medication is given as a tablet underneath the tongue, a paste or patch placed on a person's chest that allows the nitroglycerin to be absorbed through the skin, or by an IV infusion. Nitroglycerin makes the arteries and veins widen. This effect of nitroglycerin reduces the amount of work the heart has to do to meet the body's needs and may even increase the amount of blood going through the coronary arteries. Nitroglycerin also lowers blood pressure. Usually this medication's only significant side effect is to cause a headache, due to pain from blood vessels in the head widening.

In people with known CAD, the usual recommendation is to take a nitroglycerin tablet under the tongue if they have an episode of chest pain and to repeat the dose after five minutes if the pain continues. If the chest pain still hasn't gone away by five minutes after the second dose, they should take a third nitroglycerin tablet and call 911. Chest pain that doesn't go away after two nitroglycerin tablets might indeed be a heart attack.

"A" is for aspirin. This medication is given for its "blood thinning" properties. As we talked about in Chapter 5, unstable angina and heart attacks commonly involve a blood clot forming on an atherosclerotic plaque in a coronary artery, suddenly increasing the amount of blockage in it. Aspirin can help stabilize the area of the blood clot so it doesn't get worse. Aspirin may even help the body dissolve the blood clot. The usual procedure is to give the patient a standard dose of 325 mg of chewable aspirin.

All of these medications can be started "in the field" by paramedics before the patient reaches the ER. A person with chest pain who, perhaps unsure if the pain is coming from the heart or not, unwisely travels to the hospital in a car instead of an ambulance will be given these same treatments in the ER itself. A person with a suspected heart attack will also receive other medications that weren't around for our patient in 1965.

"Blood Thinners" for Heart Attacks

Besides aspirin, several other potent "blood thinners" (anticoagulants) are also routinely used in people with suspected or known heart attacks. Heparin is a blood thinner that is given as a continuous IV infusion when it is used to treat a heart attack. This medication begins working very quickly after it's started. The blood thinning effects of heparin go away rapidly if the amount of blood thinning needed must be reduced to perform certain procedures to treat a heart attack. As with any kind of blood thinner, heparin's major side effect is that it increases the risk of bleeding. Adjusting the dose of heparin so a person's blood isn't too "thin" or "thick" can be somewhat difficult, however, requiring periodic blood tests to check on this.

Newer forms of heparin—"low-molecular-weight" heparins, like enoxaparin—are given as single injections under the skin instead of through an IV line. Their dose is easier to regulate than IV heparin. However, their effects also last longer than heparin once a dose is given. If they need to be stopped to perform a procedure or if a person develops bleeding, it's more likely the patient will need to be given medication to "reverse" their blood thinning effects.

Another type of blood thinner given in the ER or soon after the patient is hospitalized, clopidogrel, can be used either with aspirin or, in patients who can't take aspirin at all, as a substitute for aspirin in patients with suspected or definite heart attacks. As we'll discuss in the next chapter, it's also a mainstay of treatment after certain heart procedures. Clopidogrel can cause bleeding, a rash, and stomach upset.

Beta-blockers and Other Medications
"Beta-blockers" are medications that decrease heart rate, lower blood pressure, and reduce how forcefully the heart contracts. All these effects decrease the amount of work the heart does, so the limited amount of oxygen a part of it is receiving due to a blockage in a coronary artery may be able to meet the heart's needs. In the ER, a beta-blocker such as metoprolol —less commonly, atenolol or propranolol—can be given intravenously so it starts working as soon as possible. One of these medications or another beta-blocker, such as carvedilol, which comes only as a pill, is then continued in an oral form.

In people who have had heart attacks, beta-blockers have been shown to reduce the risk of death and another heart attack after the patient makes it out of the hospital. Side effects from this class of medications include wheezing, fatigue, and headache. Wheezing is less likely with "cardioselective" beta-blockers like metoprolol or atenolol than it is with other beta-blockers such as propranolol. As we'll discuss in a later chapter, beta-blockers can also cause problems with sexual dysfunction. However, for our patient with a new heart attack this particular side effect is not of immediate importance.

Another class of medications, angiotensin-converting enzyme inhibitors or "ACE inhibitors," are not as commonly used in the ER to treat a heart attack. However, an ACE inhibitor is typically started in patients with heart failure and heart attacks after they are admitted to the hospital. ACE inhibitors have several beneficial effects, including reducing the pressure in both the arteries and veins—once again, decreasing the amount of work the heart has to do—and indirectly improving heart function in patients with heart failure. This class of medication reduces symptoms related to heart failure and CAD. ACE inhibitors also decrease the risk of death after hospital discharge in patients with heart attacks whose heart function is at least moderately reduced below normal.

Many different brands of ACE inhibitors are currently available, with nearly all of them used only in pill form. These include older ones like captopril, lisinopril, and enalapril, as well as newer ones like quinapril, ramipril, benazepril, and trandolapril. Potential side effects of ACE inhibitors include cough, rash, headache, and worsening kidney function. ACE inhibitors may also make blood pressure fall too much or cause an excessive increase of potassium in the blood.

"Angiotensin receptor blockers" (ARBs) are similar to ACE inhibitors. This class includes only oral medications—valsartan, candesartan, irbesartan, and several others. Their effects, indications, and side effects are similar to ACE inhibitors, with one exception. ARBs don't cause the problem with coughing that ACE inhibitors can. Thus, if a person develops a significant cough while taking an ACE inhibitor, the latter can be stopped and an ARB used instead. ACE inhibitors and ARBs can be used together for treatment of high blood pressure and some other cardiac problems.

Arrhythmias and Heart Attacks

Patients with a heart attack may also have an abnormally slow or fast heart rhythm—an "arrhythmia." Some of these abnormal heart rhythms, like ventricular fibrillation and most episodes of sustained ventricular tachycardia, are immediately life-threatening and need to be treated with an electric shock to the chest to restore normal rhythm. While our poor patient in 1965 (may he rest in peace) would have had little or no access to a defibrillator, our modern one will have many options. Besides the defibrillators present on emergency vehicles and at the hospital, many nonmedical sites (worksites, airplanes, etc.) now have a newer version available—the automatic external defibrillator (AED).

The AED is designed to be used by laypeople. If an individual collapses, a layperson trained in basic CPR can check to see if the victim is breathing and has a pulse. If the person doesn't have a pulse, due to ventricular tachycardia or ventricular fibrillation caused by a heart attack or another cause, the layperson helping the victim turns on the AED. This device then "talks through" the process of giving shocks to whoever is assisting the victim. A computer-generated voice tells this helper to put patches on the victim's bare chest and connect them to the AED. The device then analyzes the heart rhythm. If it determines the heart rhythm needs to be treated with a shock, the AED then delivers a shock automatically. It then analyzes the heart rhythm again to see if another shock is needed. The AED even warns bystanders to stay clear before each shock to prevent them from getting a shock that could hurt them. Meanwhile someone else should also be calling 911 to get more definitive help.

Abnormally slow heart rhythms can be treated either with medications like atropine that speed up the heart rate or with an "external transthoracic pacemaker." This device is different from the much smaller, permanent pacemaker a person may have implanted under the skin. (We'll talk about this type of pacemaker in a later chapter). The external transthoracic pacemaker shares much in common with the defibrillator. Both devices send electrical impulses through patches placed on the chest to the heart. In fact, they are usually combined into a single machine. However, while the defibrillator sends one big "jolt" at a time, the external pacemaker sends a series of much smaller impulses designed to stimulate the heart to beat at a certain rate.

The major downside of using an external transthoracic pacemaker is that it doesn't work on everybody. Even when it does work as designed, it can be uncomfortable for the person to get those 60 or so mild shocks through his chest every minute to keep his heart beating—although it sure beats the alternative of having no heartbeat at all! The patient can be given IV painkillers and sedatives to minimize the discomfort caused by the external transthoracic pacemaker.

An external transthoracic pacemaker can help stabilize a patient until another method for maintaining the heart rate, a "temporary transvenous pacemaker," can be used. A temporary transvenous pacemaker is a small handheld electronic device that generates electrical impulses at a rate and strength that can be adjusted over a wide range. This type of pacemaker is connected to a long, thin, plastic-coated wire inserted through a vein and placed within the right ventricle. The impulses produced by this pacemaker directly stimulate the heart to beat.

A temporary transvenous pacemaker is a more reliable and comfortable way to maintain a person's heart rate than an external transthoracic pacemaker. However, while pacing with an external transthoracic pacemaker can be started very quickly using patches placed on the chest, it takes a considerably longer time to place the special wire in the heart needed to use a temporary transvenous pacemaker. Also, this wire can be placed only by a cardiologist or other physician trained to do this procedure.

The wire needed for temporary transvenous pacing is inserted into a large vein—an internal jugular vein in the neck, a subclavian vein (located below the collarbone), or a femoral vein in the upper thigh near a person's groin. The method used to do this is called the "Seldinger technique," named after the physician who developed it, Dr. Sven-Ivar Seldinger. The skin over the vein is cleaned with an antiseptic, protected using sterile drapes, and then numbed with a local anesthetic. The vein is then punctured with a needle and a very thin, flexible wire called a "guidewire" is partially inserted into the vein. A plastic sheath or "introducer" is threaded over the guidewire and into the vein. The guidewire is removed and the pacemaker wire—more technically called a "lead"—is inserted into the vein.

This wire is threaded back to the right atrium and through the tricuspid valve until its tip is in the far end (apex) of the right ventricle. A fluoroscopy (X-ray) machine is used to see where the pacemaker wire is at any time in the patient's body and make sure it's going where it should. Some types of pacemaker wires have an inflatable balloon on the end. This balloon is inflated after the tip of the wire gets to the right atrium to help it "float" with the normal flow of blood through the tricuspid valve into the right ventricle.

Once the tip of the wire is in position within the right ventricle, the outside end of the wire is connected to the pacemaker. This device is turned on and the rate and strength of the electrical impulses it generates are adjusted to maintain a good heart rate. Since these impulses are going directly into the heart muscle through the wire, their strength is much less than the ones needed with an external transthoracic pacemaker, which has to send electrical impulses through skin, bone, and lung to reach the heart. The pacing wire will eventually be removed if the patient's own heart rate recovers, or if the patient gets a "permanent" transvenous pacemaker—more about this in Chapter 10.

"Antiarrhythmic" medications can be also be used to reduce the chance of a person developing ventricular tachycardia or ventricular fibrillation. Back when Henry did his cardiology training, it was standard procedure to use one of these medications for many (if not most) people who were hospitalized with a heart attack to prevent one of these life-threatening ventricular arrhythmias from occurring. Now these medications are reserved for people who have a continuous episode of ventricular tachycardia that is not fast enough to require a shock right away. Antiarrhythmics are also used on patients who have been successfully shocked out of ventricular tachycardia or fibrillation to try to prevent one of these life-threatening arrhythmias from happening again.

Several of these antiarrhythmic medications, such as lidocaine and procainamide, were actually available for our patient in 1965. However, one of our most important antiarrhythmic medications, amiodarone, was not. Amiodarone can be given as a continuous infusion through a vein and works quickly to prevent serious arrhythmias such as ventricular tachycardia. Amiodarone can also be given as a pill to suppress a wide variety of arrhythmias, including atrial fibrillation and ventricular tachycardia. However, it can take up to several weeks for amiodarone to reach its peak effectiveness when taken as a pill. While it doesn't usually have any serious side effects when given for a few hours or days, amiodarone has many potential side effects when it's given for a long time. Amiodarone can injure the lungs and liver, make the function of the thyroid gland abnormally high or low, and make the skin sensitive to sunlight or even turn it a blue-gray color.

Evaluation of Chest Pain

People who come to the ER are evaluated to see if their chest pain or other symptoms are due to a possible heart attack or unstable angina ("acute coronary syndrome"), or if their chest pain is due to problems with another part of the body like the lungs, bones, stomach, etc. There are three major ways this is done. The first one is a "clinical assessment" of the patient. This means the doctor, nurse, or other medical professional obtains a history from the patient and does a physical examination. People with known heart disease, the elderly, those resuscitated from ventricular fibrillation, and individuals who give a classic history of unstable or prolonged angina are likely to have chest pain that really is coming from the heart. Abnormally low blood pressure or heart rate, or abnormal heart and lung sounds suggesting congestive heart failure or other serious problems, also indicate the heart is the likely culprit and that the person needs to be hospitalized.

Second, a variety of blood tests—"cardiac enzymes"—can be done to quickly determine if the person has had any recent damage to the heart to indicate an actual or impending heart attack. None of these blood tests was either used for this purpose in 1965 or was even available then. Several of the blood tests used to check for a new or recent heart attack when Henry was in training—the SGOT and the LDH isoenzymes—have already become obsolete for diagnosing a new heart attack. Other tests, like the total creatine phosphokinase (CPK) and CPK-MB tests, were once the "gold standard" for checking whether a person is having a heart attack. Now the CPK and CPK-MB tests have been downgraded to secondary importance by newer blood tests, the troponin T and especially the troponin I. Several other blood tests, such as the serum myoglobin and CPK isoforms, are "niche" players that may be helpful for identifying heart damage several hours earlier than the other, major tests.

All of these blood tests detect the presence of chemicals released by damaged heart muscle cells. Many medical problems, such as severe infection or lack of oxygen in the blood from lung problems, can also cause a small amount of heart damage and make these tests abnormal. However, by far the most common reason most of these tests become abnormal is an actual or threatened heart attack. Generally speaking, the peak blood levels of these chemicals are proportional to the amount of heart muscle damaged. In other words, a small amount of damage to heart muscle causes a small rise in blood levels of these chemicals, while a large amount of damage causes a large rise.

An exception to this rule occurs if there is "reperfusion" of a blocked coronary artery. This means the blood clot blocking the coronary artery is removed either spontaneously by a person's own body, or by use of certain medications (such as thrombolytic agents) and procedures (like coronary angioplasty) we'll discuss later. Reperfusion allows these chemicals released by damaged heart muscle to get into the bloodstream quicker and in larger amounts than they normally would. This makes blood levels of these chemicals higher than they normally would be based on the amount of heart muscle damaged. This could make the amount of heart damaged seem greater than it actually is.

These blood tests used to check for damage to heart muscle differ in three basic ways. First, some of these tests become abnormal after a heart attack occurs sooner than others do. The level of myoglobin in blood begins to rise above normal about two hours after a heart attack starts. Myoglobin reaches its peak value about six to eight hours following a heart attack. Blood levels of troponin I and troponin T don't begin to rise above normal until about three to six hours after a heart attack begins. These troponin values don't reach their peak until about twelve hours after the heart attack. CPK and CPK-MB usually become abnormal slightly before tropinin values do. CPK and CPK-MB reach their peak values about twelve to twenty-four hours after the heart attack begins.

Second, how long these tests stay abnormal also varies widely. The blood level of myoglobin falls fairly rapidly after it reaches its peak and can miss detecting a heart attack if the person delays coming to the hospital. Elevated levels of CPK and CPK-MB typically persist for about two days after a heart attack. However, troponin I can stay abnormal for about seven to ten days following a heart attack. Tropinin T can remain abnormal for as long as two weeks after a heart attack.

Finally, myoglobin, CPK, and (to a lesser extent) CPK-MB are also present in other parts of the body besides the heart, such as the muscles in the arms and legs. Damage to these other parts of the body could also cause these tests to become abnormal, making it difficult to decide whether the heart is involved or not. On the other hand, troponin I and, to mildly lesser degree, troponin T are present almost exclusively in the heart. Currently, troponin I is the "gold standard" for detecting heart damage due to its high reliability for detecting damage to the heart in a reasonably short amount of time after a heart attack.

Besides clinical assessment and these blood tests, the third way to check for a heart attack is an EKG. Patients with heart attacks are divided based on the EKG into those who have "non-ST-elevation myocardial infarction" and those with "ST-elevation myocardial infarction." The first group of people, as well as those with unstable angina, have either no or only mild, usually temporary abnormalities on their EKG. They also, at least initially, have an overall lower risk of dying than those with ST segment elevation myocardial infarction. If their chest pain goes away with the medications we've described so far, they can be admitted directly to the hospital for further evaluation and treatment. Those judged to be at lower risk are admitted to a regular hospital bed on a "telemetry" unit. The nurses working on the telemetry unit have special training in how to evaluate and treat heart problems. They monitor the patient's heart rhythm continuously on a display screen so any new problems can be identified and treated quickly.

Inside the Intensive Care Unit

Patients at higher risk can be admitted to an intensive care unit. There they can be watched more closely for recurrent chest pain or other problems. Those who develop serious problems like severe congestive heart failure or very low blood pressure can be treated with other medications or have procedures done to help them. For example, IV nitroglycerin or another medication, IV nitroprusside, can be used to decrease pressures in the heart and the arteries of the lungs in people with severe congestive heart failure and fluid in their lung tissue (pulmonary edema).

A "Swan-Ganz catheter"—a long thin plastic tube with an inflatable balloon on the end—can be inserted into a vein and passed into the right side of the heart, just like the lead for the temporary transvenous pacemaker we described previously. However, instead of staying in the right ventricle like the pacemaker lead, this catheter is threaded out through the pulmonary artery and into one of this artery's branches, usually the right pulmonary artery. The Swan-Ganz catheter measures pressures within the pulmonary artery. By blowing up the balloon at its end temporarily, the catheter can also measure a "wedge" pressure—the diastolic pressure in the left ventricle. If these pressures are too high, medications such as IV nitroglycerin or ones that remove excess fluid from the body (diuretics) can help to lower them.

The Swan-Ganz catheter can also identify people whose heart function is so low they need additional medicines to stimulate the heart. Dobutamine is given through a vein and increases how forcefully the heart contracts. At low doses another IV medication, dopamine, also stimulates the heart. At higher doses, dopamine acts mainly by making arteries constrict and can help raise blood pressure when it is too low. Another IV medication, norepinephrine, is used exclusively to increase blood pressure when it is dangerously low.

An "intra-aortic balloon pump" is a device that can be used to support a person with low blood pressure and reduce the amount of work the heart has to do. Like another procedure we'll discuss soon, coronary angiography, it involves inserting a catheter into an artery in the groin and advancing it into the aorta. However, this catheter is somewhat thicker and has a large long inflatable balloon on its end. The tip of the catheter is positioned in the aorta just before the left subclavian artery—the artery that supplies blood to the left arm—comes off it.

The end of the catheter outside the body is connected to a pump that makes the balloon inflate and deflate in a continuous cycle with every heartbeat. The balloon inflates during diastole, when the aortic valve is closed. This helps force more blood into the arteries of the heart. The balloon deflates during systole, when the aortic valve is open and the left ventricle is pumping blood out into the aorta. When the balloon deflates it allows blood to pass through the aorta to the rest of the body. Balloon deflation also produces a kind of mild "suction" effect that reduces the amount of resistance to blood flow, thus helping the heart to pump more blood out to the rest of the body with less work.

The effects of the intra-aortic balloon pump on the heart and coronary arteries can be beneficial for people with a variety of serious heart problems. These include people with severely decreased heart function, those with severe coronary artery disease, and those with certain complications of a heart attack we'll discuss later, such as sudden and severe mitral regurgitation.

Thrombolytic Treatment and Coronary Angiography
Patients with ST-elevation myocardial infarction need more than just medicine before they can be tucked into a hospital bed for the night. They are likely to have a blocked coronary artery that, as time passes, will cause more and more heart muscle to die. It's critical that the artery be opened up as soon as possible to restore blood flow and prevent as much further damage to the heart muscle (myocardium) as possible. The rule is, "Time is myocardium."

One way to do this has been used since the middle of the 1980s. Thrombolytic therapy involves giving a medication that "dissolves" the blood clot in a blocked artery. The patient is given an IV dose of streptokinase or, more likely, one of the newer thrombolytic agents such as alteplase, reteplase, or tenecteplase. Other medications used to treat the blood clot, like aspirin and heparin, are also given. The combination of these medications will at least partially open the blocked artery in a significant number of people. Even giving these thrombolytic agents as long as 12 hours after a heart attack begins can be beneficial.

Thrombolytic therapy had a brief reign as the preferred way to treat patients with ST-elevation myocardial infarction. However, it's now been relegated to being the "backup" for a better therapy—actually going in and opening up the blocked artery. Doing this requires performing a "coronary angiogram." This procedure can be done on a person with a heart attack to see if CAD is present. As we'll discuss in a later chapter, coronary angiography can also be done in stable patients suspected of having CAD, as well as those with known CAD that is causing more chest pain or other problems. A cardiologist needs specialized training to perform coronary angiography.

Coronary angiography involves inserting a long narrow tube called a catheter into an artery. Either the femoral artery, located in the upper thigh near the groin, or an artery in the arm can be used for coronary angiography. The catheter is inserted into the artery using the Seldinger technique, the method we described earlier that's used to insert the wire needed for temporary transvenous pacing into a vein. During coronary angiography the artery is punctured with a needle and a long thin wire is inserted into it. A catheter that is about as long and slightly wider than this wire is threaded over it into the artery.

As the cardiologist watches it using a fluoroscopy machine, the catheter is advanced into the artery and then back through the aorta until it reaches the heart itself. After the wire is removed the tip of the catheter is inserted into the opening of a coronary artery and X-ray contrast ("dye") is injected into the artery. Movies taken using the fluoroscopy machine show how the contrast flows through the artery. A "pinched" area where the flow of contrast looks narrowed, or an area where the contrast stops flowing entirely, indicates the presence of a blockage.

If a coronary artery is severely or completely blocked, the cardiologist usually tries to open it up using any of several different methods. In a person having a heart attack due to a fresh blood clot in a coronary artery, the cardiologist may try to create a tiny opening in the clot with the guide wire or infuse a low dose of a thrombolytic medication through the catheter into the blocked artery. Eventually the cardiologist will try to do a procedure called coronary angioplasty (or, occasionally, a similar type of procedure) that widens the artery and lets more blood get through it. Coronary angioplasty is performed by placing a special catheter with an inflatable balloon at the end into an area of blockage in a coronary artery. Inflating the balloon reduces the amount of blockage in the artery. We'll discuss coronary angioplasty and similar procedures in more detail in Chapter 10.

During this procedure the cardiologist also uses another type of catheter to perform a "cardiac catheterization." This catheter is used to check for any abnormal pressures within the left ventricle, or a significant fall in pressure across the aortic valve from the left ventricle to the aorta that indicates the presence of aortic stenosis. This catheter also injects contrast into the left ventricle to see how well its walls contract and if there is significant mitral regurgitation.

As with any procedure in which something is placed inside the body, coronary angiography does carry a small level of risk. Serious complications such as stroke, heart attack, or death can occur. Fortunately, these complications are rare. Damage to the artery used for the procedure or excessive bleeding from the artery occurs occasionally. The X-ray contrast injected into the coronary arteries can also cause reactions ranging from hives to, rarely, death. The contrast can also occasionally worsen kidney function, especially in people with diabetes—an effect that is usually only temporary but can be permanent.

Coronary angiography is indicated as "first-line" treatment in patients identified as having an ST-elevation myocardial infarction that started within the previous 12 hours, and sometimes longer, such as if the person is still having chest pain. This assumes, however, that coronary angiography and angioplasty can be done within about 90 minutes after the patient reaches the hospital. Sometimes this can't be done. For example, not all hospitals have the facilities and specially trained cardiologists and nurses needed to do coronary angiography. If the person can't be transferred to a hospital that does coronary angiography and coronary angioplasty and have the latter procedure done within that "window" of 90 minutes, then the best alternative is to give thrombolytic therapy. The patient can then be transferred to a hospital that performs coronary angiography and evaluated regarding when or if that procedure still needs to be done.

Sometimes the thrombolytic medication doesn't help and the patient is still having chest pain. In that case, "rescue" coronary angiography and angioplasty can be done at the other hospital. However, if the patient "cools down"—the person's chest pain goes away, the EKG doesn't show anymore that the heart is not getting enough blood, and the individual is now stable—coronary angiography isn't done right away. Depending on how the patient does, however, this procedure may be done later. Coronary angiography is preferably delayed for at least 24 hours after the thrombolytic medication was given, after its blood thinning effects have worn off.

Our poor modern man with the heart attack has been through a lot already. Let's tuck him in for the night and give him a chance to rest. We'll continue our discussion of how to treat a heart attack in the next chapter.

Chapter 7 Summary

- ♥ Evaluation and treatment of a heart attack has improved dramatically in recent decades.

- ♥ Initial assessment of a person with a suspected heart attack includes a history and physical examination, cardiac enzymes, and an electrocardiogram (EKG).

- ♥ Medications used to treat a heart attack include those that help "dissolve" a blood clot in a blocked coronary artery, relieve chest pain, and reduce the amount of work done by the heart.

- ♥ Defibrillators are used to treat certain abnormal, life-threatening heart rhythms caused by a heart attack. Pacemakers are used to treat serious slow heart rhythms.

- ♥ Coronary angiography is used to look for coronary artery disease in most people with a heart attack.

Chapter 8: High-Tech Heart Tests
Evaluating Risks to Your Heart

Chapter Preview:
Modern Stress Tests
    Exercise stress tests
Echocardiography
    Transthoracic echocardiogram
    Doppler study
    Transesophageal echocardiogram
Myocardial Perfusion Imaging
    Thallium-201 and technetium-99m agents
    Fixed and reversible defects
Pharmacologic Stress Testing
    Dobutamine stress test
    Dipyridamole and adenosine stress tests
Complications of a Heart Attack
    Partial or complete rupture of a papillary muscle
    Ventricular septal defect
    Rupture of the heart and pseudoaneurysm
    "True" aneurysm
    Dressler syndrome
Home from the Hospital
    Medications used after a heart attack
    Lifestyle instructions

REMEMBER OUR MAN with the heart attack in 1965? Back then there was little that could be done to assess his risk of having more chest pain or suffering another heart attack. Techniques for performing coronary angiography were just starting to be developed, and this test wasn't routinely available or done in 1965. Instead, our patient might have a simple type of "stress test" before he went home from the hospital. The

Master's two-step test involved having a person repeatedly walk up and down a wooden structure consisting of two steps—hence the "two-step" part of the test's name. The heart rate and blood pressure were checked and an EKG (electrocardiogram) was taken before and after this walking to see if there was evidence the heart wasn't getting enough blood—"myocardial ischemia." The patient was also asked whether or not any chest pain occurred during the test.

Unfortunately, the Master's two-step test often failed to identify people at risk for further heart problems. Even if the test did show a person had myocardial ischemia, the major medications and procedures like coronary angioplasty that are now used to treat it were still years or even decades away.

Modern Stress Tests

Modern patients initially thought to be at low and, in some cases, moderate risk of further heart problems after a heart attack or unstable angina may also have a stress test to "risk stratify" them. The stress test is done to get a better idea if they really are at reasonably low risk for a future heart attack or death due to their heart disease, or if they have evidence the heart is still having problems and they need a coronary angiogram. The kinds of stress tests done today use considerably more sophisticated technology and are much more helpful than the one our man in 1965 might have performed. These modern stress tests are most commonly performed for reasons other than evaluating a person shortly after a heart attack. For example, these tests can evaluate patients with chest pain to see if they have evidence of exercise-induced myocardial ischemia caused by coronary artery disease (CAD). Patients already known to have CAD can perform a stress test to see if they require any additional medications or procedures to treat their CAD.

The usual type of modern stress test involves having a person do increasing levels of exercise while the EKG, heart rate, and blood pressure are monitored. A stationary bicycle can be used. However, exercise is usually done on a treadmill. The treadmill starts at a low speed. The treadmill periodically gets faster and steeper at intervals ranging from seconds to several minutes. Usually the person doing the test is asked to exercise until he or she needs to stop due to shortness of breath, chest pain, or other problems, or until a certain heart rate and blood pressure is reached to make sure the heart is stressed enough. Sometimes, especially soon after a heart attack, only a "submaximal" stress test is done. This means the stress test is stopped at a moderate level of exertion or increase in heart rate, even though the person wasn't too tired to stop yet and could have walked longer.

A person may develop chest pain during the exercise test. With the exception of someone who's had a recent heart attack, having chest pain is not by itself a reliable sign the person has significant CAD. In fact, most people who have CAD won't have chest pain during the test. Others may have chest pain that is really coming from their stomach, lungs, muscles, or other part of their body and has nothing to do with their heart.

The EKG is more useful for seeing if the heart isn't getting enough blood with exercise than whether or not a person has chest pain. The EKG will show changes that indicate the heart is not getting enough blood in about 60% of people with CAD. However, using the EKG alone to see if a person's heart is not getting enough blood has its own limitations. The EKG won't identify about 40% of people with CAD. In some individuals, especially young women and those taking certain medicines like digoxin, the EKG may show changes with exercise that mimic those seen in patients with CAD, even though the person doesn't really have this problem. This same "false positive" result may also occur if the EKG shows certain types of abnormalities—problems with the way the heart conducts electricity, increased thickness of the heart muscle, etc.—before the person starts to exercise.

Adding a test that takes pictures of the heart—an "imaging test"—before and after exercise increases the chance of identifying someone with CAD to about 90%. An imaging test can also be less likely than the EKG to indicate a person has CAD when this disease isn't really present. There are two standard ways to take pictures of the heart with an exercise test: echocardiography and myocardial perfusion imaging.

Echocardiography
An echocardiogram, or "echo" for short, involves sending an ultrasound beam through the person's chest using a handheld probe (transducer). As its name suggests the ultrasound beam consists of sound waves. However, these sound waves are at a frequency over 100 times higher than we can hear. An echocardiogram doesn't involve any type of radiation like you would get with an X-ray and causes no harm to the patient.

The ultrasound beam produced by the transducer bounces off the walls, valves, and other parts of the heart. The transducer then picks up these "echoes." The echocardiogram machine processes the signals based on how strong the echo signals are and how long it took them to return to the transducer after bouncing off a wall or other part of the heart. The information obtained is displayed on a TV screen as still pictures or like a movie. The echocardiogram is useful for seeing how well the heart is contracting and evaluating the heart valves. It can see if the heart chambers are enlarged and checks for increased fluid around the heart—"pericardial effusion." The echocardiogram can also identify any masses like blood clots or tumors within the heart.

Besides obtaining these pictures of the heart, an echocardiogram machine is used to obtain a "Doppler study." This uses ultrasound signals to measure the velocity of blood flow in different areas of the heart. "Color flow Doppler" displays this information about how blood is moving through the heart as moving colors on a TV screen. A Doppler study is routinely used in people with aortic or mitral stenosis to see how badly their valve is narrowed, since blood moves at higher velocities as the degree of narrowing gets worse. A Doppler study is also used to check for increased stiffness of the left ventricle, which could potentially cause heart failure.

Sometimes an echocardiogram done in the usual way, with the probe on a person's chest ("transthoracic" echocardiogram), may not give pictures that are good enough to evaluate the heart. This problem is more likely to occur in people who are overweight or have lung disease, like emphysema. These conditions increase the distance and amount of air between the probe and the heart, weakening the ultrasound beam. Also, some areas of the heart aren't usually seen at all on a transthoracic echocardiogram. This includes a small "pouch" that comes off the left atrium called the left atrial appendage. Blood clots can form in the left atrial appendage, especially in patients with atrial fibrillation and mitral stenosis. Seeing whether or not there is a blood clot is in the left atrial appendage can make a big difference in deciding what treatment is best for a person.

In these circumstances, a "transesophageal" echocardiogram can be done. The person's throat is sprayed with an anesthetic to numb it. Intravenous medication is given to make the patient drowsy. A long hose-like probe is then placed in the back of the person's throat and swallowed. The probe passes into the esophagus, the tube that connects the throat to the stomach, and is positioned behind the heart. Transducers at the end of the probe then take ultrasound pictures and do a Doppler study.

A transesophageal echocardiogram produces sharper and clearer pictures of the heart than those typically obtained with a transthoracic echocardiogram. This is because the transducer is right next to the heart and the ultrasound beam can reach it more easily. It also means that subtle abnormalities that couldn't be seen on the usual type of echocardiogram, like vegetations—abnormal material on an infected heart valve—or small blood clots, can be easily identified on a transesophageal echocardiogram. Areas that are difficult or impossible to see on a transthoracic echocardiogram, such as the left atrial appendage and most of the aorta within the chest, are also easily evaluated with a transesophageal echocardiogram.

A transthoracic echocardiogram is usually done by a special technologist—"sonographer"—alone and carries virtually no risk to the patient. On the other hand, a transesophageal echocardiogram needs to be done by a cardiologist or another physician specially trained to do this procedure, assisted by a technologist who runs the echocardiogram machine. A transesophageal echocardiogram is also more uncomfortable for the patient and does carry a very small amount of risk. Serious complications such as bleeding, infection, or injury to the esophagus can occur, but they are rare.

Since it is used to evaluate so many potential problems with the heart, a resting echocardiogram is often done as a separate test, without the person exercising. When done with a stress test, the echocardiogram is performed before the person exercises, with special views obtained to see how well the left ventricle is contracting. If the whole left ventricle is not contracting well or if only part of it isn't, this is suspicious by itself for possible CAD even without doing the stress test. If the person walks on a treadmill, new pictures of the heart are taken immediately after exercise ends. If a stationary bicycle is used, pictures of the heart can be taken with the echocardiogram machine while the person is still pedaling on the bicycle.

The left ventricle normally responds to exercise by contracting harder. The stress test is abnormal if the echocardiogram shows an area of the heart that is not contracting as hard immediately after exercise as it did before the person started the test. This response strongly implies the area of the heart wasn't getting enough blood during exercise and that there is a blockage in the artery supplying blood to it.

Since it's so important to be able to see the left ventricle well both before and after a stress test, sometimes a person is injected with a "contrast agent" to improve the quality of the pictures obtained with the echocardiogram. The material used in this type of contrast agent is entirely different than the X-ray contrast used for a coronary angiogram. The contrast agent consists of tiny bubbles and is injected into a vein before images of the left ventricle are taken. It passes through the right side of the heart and the blood vessels of the lungs to reach the left ventricle. The contrast agent helps identify the inner lining of the left ventricle to see if this ventricle is contracting and thickening as well as it should. The tiny bubbles in the contrast agent are broken down and cleared by the body within minutes.

Myocardial Perfusion Imaging
The other method for taking pictures of the heart with a stress test is myocardial perfusion imaging (MPI). While the echocardiogram gives a good general overview of what's going on with the heart, MPI specializes in seeing if any areas of the heart are not getting enough blood or have been damaged. This test involves injecting a small amount of "low-level" (mildly) radioactive material into an arm vein. Several types of radioactive material can be used. The most common "radiotracers" used are thallium-201 and technetium-99m. Technetium-99m is combined with a material that is not radioactive. Technetium-99m is usually given in the form of technetium-99m sestamibi (Cardiolite) or technetium-99m tetrofosmin (Myoview).

These radiotracers work by going to areas of the heart where there is good blood flow and where the heart muscle cells are functioning. If an area of the heart has been damaged previously, or if it is temporarily not getting enough blood, not as much of the radioactive material will go to that area. A special camera that detects the radioactivity produced by these materials takes images of the heart. These images show if any areas of the heart aren't getting enough blood or have been damaged. Nowadays, the images of the heart are usually obtained using a technique called "single-photon emission computed tomography" or SPECT.

A stress test done with MPI has two parts. When thallium-201 is used by itself, it is injected into a vein about a minute or two before the person reaches the peak level of exercise. Images of the heart are then taken about 10 to 15 minutes after the exercise test is finished. A second set of heart images is obtained about 3 to 4 hours later. Images taken just after the stress test are compared to those taken hours later.

An area of the heart that shows abnormally low uptake of the radiotracer on both sets of images is a "fixed defect." It can mean that part of the heart has been damaged before, such as from a heart attack. An area that looks abnormal on the images taken right after the stress test but shows significantly more radiotracer activity on the second set of images is a "reversible" defect. A reversible defect strongly suggests that there's a blockage in a coronary artery that's bad enough to give the heart less blood than it needs when a person is exercising. However, there's still enough blood flow through the blockage for the thallium-201 to slowly get into the abnormal area of the heart by several hours after the exercise test. It also means the person needs further evaluation and treatment because he or she is at increased risk for a heart attack.

When either technetium-99m sestamibi or technetium-99m tetrofosmin is used, two separate imaging studies are done. "Rest" images are obtained after a person is injected with one of these two technetium-99m agents while sitting quietly and not exercising. "Stress" images are obtained shortly after the person is injected with the technetium-99m agent about one or two minutes before finishing an exercise test. Either the rest images or stress images can be obtained first. The rest study and the stress study can even be done on two separate days. The rest and stress images are compared to look for fixed or reversible defects.

A "gated" study can also be done to see how well each wall of the left ventricle contracts and to evaluate the left ventricle's overall systolic function. "Gated" means the EKG is used to time the taking of separate pictures of the heart as it contracts during different phases of systole. These pictures, usually eight to sixteen in number, are combined into a short repeating "movie" that shows the heart contracting during an "average" heartbeat.

Instead of using just one type of radioactive material to evaluate blood flow to the heart, a "dual-isotope" study can be performed instead. This test begins with a rest study using thallium-201. About an hour or so later a stress test is done with either technetium-99m sestamibi or technetium-99m tetrofosmin. The rest and stress images are then reviewed and compared to see if there are any areas of the heart not getting enough blood or possibly damaged.

Besides helping to determine if a person has CAD, myocardial perfusion imaging provides important information for predicting the risk of having serious heart problems in the future. A person who has an exercise test with normal myocardial perfusion images has, in general, a risk of having a heart attack or dying from a heart-related cause that is less than 1% over the next year. The risk of these events over the next year is 7% or more in someone who has an exercise test with very abnormal myocardial perfusion images.

Although used less frequently than in the past, another type of test done to evaluate the heart using technetium-99m is a "radionuclide ventriculogram." This test is used to assess the function of the left ventricle and the right ventricle. It can be done either by itself or as part of an exercise stress test. A person's red blood cells are "tagged" or labeled with technetium-99m so that a nuclear camera can see the blood within the heart. This test is very accurate for measuring the "ejection fraction" of the left ventricle and right ventricle—the percentage of blood pumped out of either ventricle when it contracts during systole.

Pharmacologic Stress Testing

For an exercise test to reliably check if someone has CAD the person must be able to walk long enough on a treadmill and get the heart rate high enough to make sure the heart is being "stressed" as much as it should. The goal is to reach 85 to 100% of the "age-predicted maximal heart rate." This is the maximum heart rate a person is expected to reach based on his or her age. The age-predicted maximum heart rate decreases as a person gets older. This maximum heart rate is estimated by taking 220 and subtracting the person's age in years.

Some people can't walk well enough on a treadmill to increase their heart rate and stress their heart enough. This can be due to arthritis in their legs, shortness of breath caused by lung disease or other health problems, etc. These people can have an alternative form of stress test that doesn't require vigorous walking. They receive one of two different types of medication as part of a "pharmacologic" stress test.

One of the medications used for a pharmacologic stress test, dobutamine, stimulates the heart and increases the heart rate, like exercise does. However, while blood pressure normally goes up with exercise, blood pressure may go either up or down with dobutamine. This medication is given at increasing doses through a vein. The effects of dobutamine wear off within minutes once the test is over and the dobutamine infusion is stopped.

Sometimes an additional medicine, atropine, is given intravenously to increase the heart rate if the dobutamine doesn't raise heart rate enough by itself. As with an exercise test, the goal is to increase the heart rate to between 85 and 100% of the age-predicted maximal heart rate. Certain medications, like beta-blockers, block the effects of dobutamine and make it more difficult to do the test. Side effects of dobutamine include palpitations, feeling anxious, and nausea. However, these side effects go away quickly after dobutamine is stopped.

Adenosine and dipyridamole are two similar medications given intravenously that work differently from dobutamine. Unlike exercise or dobutamine, they usually cause little change in heart rate or blood pressure. Instead they make the arteries of the heart widen and increase blood flow to the heart. An artery with a significant blockage doesn't widen as much as a normal artery. A stress test using adenosine or dipyridamole detects the lower amount of blood flow in an abnormal artery compared to normal ones. Both adenosine and dipyridamole can cause side effects such as shortness of breath, wheezing, and lightheadedness that go away after the medication is stopped. Another medication, aminophylline, can be given intravenously to treat side effects of dipyridamole such as wheezing. A person should also not eat or drink anything containing caffeine, such as coffee or tea, for at least 12 hours before having an adenosine or dipyridamole stress test. This is because caffeine interferes with adenosine and dipyridamole and can make the stress test appear normal even if a person really does have CAD.

Pharmacologic stress tests using dobutamine, adenosine, or dipyridamole require that pictures be taken of the heart. The EKG is significantly less likely to show if the heart is not getting enough blood with these tests than it is with an exercise test, especially when adenosine or dipyridamole are used. However, by using MPI or an echocardiogram with these pharmacologic stress tests, the chance of detecting CAD is about the same as when these pictures are taken with an exercise test.

Although it can be used with MPI, dobutamine stress tests are usually done with an echocardiogram. On the other hand, adenosine and dipyridamole stress tests are usually combined with MPI. Another difference is that a dobutamine stress test is done with the person not exercising at all. Although not absolutely necessary, it's better if a person can perform a low, steady level of walking on a treadmill while he's having an adenosine or dipyridamole stress test. Doing this improves the quality of the pictures taken of the heart and may also reduce the chances of the person having side effects.

Complications of a Heart Attack
While he's in the hospital and having all these tests done, our modern patient with a heart attack will be watched for any further serious problems. A small percentage of people will have late complications after a heart attack, such as problems with slow or fast abnormal heart rhythms. His heart rhythm will be monitored to check for any of these problems.

Several serious complications can occur due to damage to certain parts of the heart after a heart attack. One of the small muscles—"papillary muscles"— that help attach the mitral valve leaflets to the left ventricle can partially or completely rupture. This prevents the mitral valve from closing normally and causes severe leaking or "regurgitation" of the valve. Complete rupture of a papillary muscle usually causes death quickly. Partial rupture of one of these muscles may not be immediately life-threatening, but it can cause heart failure serious enough to eventually cause death.

A heart attack can also cause a rupture in the tissue separating the right ventricle and the left ventricle, the interventricular septum. This creates a "ventricular septal defect," with abnormal blood flow from the left ventricle to the right ventricle. Depending on the size of the rupture, a ventricular septal defect can cause heart failure and death within hours to days.

The heart itself may rupture after a heart attack. The area of the heart that ruptures is usually in the left ventricle, near the boundary between damaged and normal heart muscle. Rupture of the heart causes bleeding into the space that separates the heart from the thin tissue that surrounds it like a bag, the pericardium. The blood going into this pericardial space causes a "hemopericardium." This blood can compress the heart so much it can't work well enough to sustain life.

Sometimes this blood may clot and seal off the ruptured area of the heart. Eventually this can produce a "pseudoaneurysm." A pseudoaneurysm is an area of bulging where the heart ruptured. It contains blood clots surrounded by a "pouch" of pericardial tissue. Blood can flow between the left ventricle and into the pseudoaneurysm with each beat through a narrow "neck" connecting the cavity of the left ventricle with the pseudoaneurysm. Blood clots in the pseudoaneurysm can break off and travel to other parts of the body, causing a stroke or other damage. Sometimes, even days or months after a heart attack, the pseudoaneurysm itself may rupture and cause death. When a pseudoaneurysm is found, surgery is recommended to treat it.

The unfortunate people who have rupture of a papillary muscle, the interventricular septum, or the heart itself usually do it within the first week after a heart attack. Each of these three problems can cause a person to suddenly become short of breath and make the blood pressure fall. A new heart murmur, indicating abnormal blood flow, is present in about nine out of ten people who develop a ventricular septal defect and about half of those who have rupture of a papillary muscle. An echocardiogram is used to check if a rupture of any of these three areas is present.

Rupture of a papillary muscle, the interventricular septum, or the heart itself carries a very high risk of death. For each one of these complications, surgery to treat the problem can significantly decrease the chance of dying. However, although the risk of dying during or after an operation is usually lower than if surgery isn't done, the risk of death with surgery itself is still significant.

Another problem that can occur after a heart attack is a left ventricular aneurysm. An aneurysm is caused by the damaged area of the heart becoming thin and bulging out from the rest of the heart. The aneurysm forms a "pocket" that doesn't contract and pump blood. Unlike a pseudoaneurysm, a "true" aneurysm is not caused by rupture of the heart. Its wall consists of heart muscle and scar tissue rather than pericardium. While a pseudoaneurysm has a significant chance of eventually rupturing, a true aneurysm rarely ruptures.

A left ventricular aneurysm can cause several serious problems. It doesn't contract and pump blood like the rest of the left ventricle. This can reduce overall heart function. Also, blood can "pool" inside the left ventricular aneurysm and form blood clots. These blood clots can break off and cause strokes and damage other parts of the body. Warfarin, a blood thinner taken by mouth, can be used to reduce the chance of this happening. A left ventricular aneurysm can also increase a person's odds of having abnormal, potentially life-threatening heart rhythms such as ventricular tachycardia. Sometimes surgery to remove the aneurysm is needed.

Dressler syndrome can occur about one week to two months after a heart attack. It is caused by inflammation of the pericardium. A person may have sharp chest pains, fever, and fluid around the heart. Dressler syndrome can be treated with high doses of aspirin to reduce pain and inflammation.

Home from the Hospital

Assuming that everything goes well in the hospital, a person will go home after a heart attack with certain standard medications. These include aspirin, a beta-blocker, and nitroglycerin tablets to put under the tongue for any future chest pains. People whose left ventricular systolic function is at least moderately decreased after a heart attack are also given an ACE inhibitor. Other medications may be substituted for these ones if a person can't tolerate a particular medicine due to side effects. For example, a person may get a bad cough with ACE inhibitors. In that case, an angiotensin receptor blocker (ARB) might be used instead. ARBs have beneficial effects similar to ACE inhibitors except they don't cause cough.

Another blood thinner we talked about before, clopidogrel, is also very likely to be in this mix. Sometimes other types of heart medications will also be used in particular situations—more about this later.

While in the hospital, our modern man or woman with a heart attack will also have blood tests done to check for abnormal kidney and liver function, abnormal levels of minerals like potassium in the blood, elevated blood sugar that could be caused by diabetes, and blood counts to look for anemia and other problems. This person will also have the cholesterol level checked. It is very likely this individual will be sent home on one of the cholesterol-lowering medications we'll talk about later. Someone who is a smoker will be helped to quit this habit. Blood pressure will be monitored throughout the stay in the hospital. If necessary, our heart attack victim will be given medications to treat high blood pressure.

Our modern person will also be given instructions about exercise and diet before leaving the hospital. These instructions will include details about how much and how long a person should exercise based on the severity of heart disease present and the individual's overall health. Recommendations will also be given about the maximum number of calories a person should eat every day and what kinds of food to eat to restrict the total amount of cholesterol and salt in the person's diet to a healthy level.

The doctor will usually wait about three to four weeks after a person has a heart attack to decide when it is safe for this individual to return to work. An exercise stress test is sometimes done about that time to see if a patient is up to the demands of going back to work, particularly if this person has a physically strenuous job. Most hospitals and communities also have formal cardiac rehabilitation programs. These programs typically include exercise sessions where the person can be monitored more closely for any problems with arrhythmias, chest pain, or abnormally high or low blood pressure during exercise.

Our man with the heart attack in 1965 would be advised to do little or no activity for weeks or months after a heart attack. However, our modern heart attack survivor will be encouraged to become active and exercise as soon as possible. Among its other beneficial effects, exercise makes a person's muscles work more efficiently. When the muscles work better the heart has to do less work to supply them with blood.

We'll talk about when a particularly important kind of exercise, sex, can resume after a heart attack in Chapter 12.

Chapter 8 Summary

- ♥ Stress tests, done either with exercise or medications, are used to evaluate people with known or suspected coronary artery disease.

- ♥ Echocardiography is used to evaluate the heart's function and valves either as a separate test or as part of a stress test.

- ♥ Myocardial perfusion imaging uses "low-level" (mildly) radioactive materials to help determine if a person has coronary artery disease and to estimate the risk of having a heart attack or dying from any heart-related cause.

♥ Serious complications of a heart attack include partial or complete rupture of a papillary muscle causing mitral regurgitation; ventricular septal defect; and rupture of the heart.

♥ Medications commonly prescribed following a heart attack include aspirin, nitroglycerin, beta-blockers, angiotensin-converting enzyme inhibitors, angiotensin receptor blockers, and statins or other medicines used to lower cholesterol.

Chapter 9: More Tests and Treatments
Managing and Medicating Heart and Blood Vessel Disease

Chapter Preview:
At the Doctor's Office
    The history and physical
    Blood tests
    EKG and chest X-ray
Tests for Arrhythmias
    Holter monitor
    Event monitor
    Insertable loop recorder
    Tilt table test
    Electrophysiology study
Magnetic Resonance Imaging and Computed Tomography
    Assessment of abnormalities in the heart and arteries
    Evaluating calcium and blockages in the coronary arteries
Tests for Arterial Disease
    MRI, CT scanning, and ultrasound
    Ankle-brachial index
    Arteriograms
Medications for Heart Disease
    Beta-blockers
    ACE inhibitors and angiotensin receptor blockers
    Nitrates
    Calcium antagonists
    Diuretics
    Digoxin
    Ranolazine
    Antiarrhythmics

Antihypertensives
Cholesterol-lowering medications
Cardiology in the Future
Future tests and treatments

THE BEST WAY to treat a heart attack is to prevent one from happening in the first place. A person who has chest pain, shortness of breath, or other symptoms that could be due to heart problems should see his or her doctor and be checked out before the "big one" occurs. The same holds true for any of the other possible heart problems we've discussed in previous chapters, such as heart failure, hypertension, valve problems, arrhythmias, etc.

At the Doctor's Office
Your doctor will obtain a good history—the story of your present and past medical problems. You'll be asked about any suspicious symptoms such as chest pain, shortness of breath, palpitations, or passing out. You'll tell your doctor whether you have any past history of heart problems as a child or adult.

It's important for your doctor to know if you have a history of high blood pressure, diabetes, high cholesterol, or have ever used tobacco. All of these risk factors increase your chance of having coronary artery disease (CAD). Having a parent, brother, or sister who developed CAD at an early age—55 years old or younger for male relatives, 65 years old or less for female relatives—also increases your risk of developing CAD if you are younger than those ages.

Your doctor also needs to know if you've ever had specific cardiac tests such as a stress test, echocardiogram, or coronary angiogram. The doctor will need to review the results of these tests to see what kinds of heart problems you've had before. These old tests can also help determine if you need additional heart tests.

Here's a very important fact to know—people with severe CAD may have a completely normal physical examination. Nonetheless, a good exam can provide your doctor with important clues as to your chances of having heart disease. Abnormally high or low blood pressure and heart rate can be picked up on the examination. Listening to the lungs can detect signs of increased fluid in them and possible heart failure. This can then be evaluated further with a chest X-ray or other tests. Your doctor will check for blockage in the arteries of your neck and legs. This can cause decreased strength of the pulses in these areas, or an abnormal "swishing" sound (called a bruit) that's heard by listening over these arteries with a stethoscope. Even looking inside the eyes with an "ophthalmoscope" can detect changes in the blood vessels there that occur with chronic hypertension and diabetes.

Your doctor will listen very carefully to your heart with a stethoscope. The technical term for this is "auscultation." The two parts of the "lub-dub" of normal heart sounds are more formally called "S_1" and "S_2." They are caused by changes in blood flow and closure of heart valves. S_1 marks the end of diastole and the beginning of systole, when the mitral and tricuspid valves close, the aortic and pulmonic valves open, and both ventricles contract. S_2 marks the end of systole and the beginning of diastole, when the mitral and tricuspid valves open, the aortic and pulmonic valves close, and both ventricles fill with blood from the two atria.

S_2 actually consists of two sounds normally heard very close together—A_2, due to closure of the aortic valve, and P_2, due to closure of the pulmonic valve. A_2 normally occurs a little before P_2. Taking a deep breath makes P_2 occur a little later and A_2 occur slightly earlier, increasing the time between when A_2 and then P_2 are heard. This is called "physiological splitting of S_2." Some kinds of heart disease can change this relationship between A_2 and P_2. For example, severe narrowing (stenosis) of the aortic valve can make A_2 occur after P_2. When a person with this problem takes a deep breath the two sounds of S_2 may be heard closer together rather than farther apart as they normally do—"reversed splitting of S_2."

Two extra sounds, S_3 and S_4, are also sometimes heard. A person with one or both of these extra heart sounds is said to have a "gallop" rhythm. A gallop may or may not be abnormal, depending on a person's age. S_3 is a low-pitched sound heard a little after S_2, early in diastole when the left ventricle and right ventricle are filling with blood from their respective atria. It is normal for children and young adults to have an S_3. In older adults, however, an S_3 is abnormal. It can be heard in people with heart failure and those with severe mitral regurgitation.

S_4 is a low-pitched sound that occurs late in diastole just before S_1, when the atria contract and push more blood into the ventricles. Unlike an S_3, an S_4 is not normally heard in children and young adults. An S_4 can be heard in some older adults without evidence of heart disease. However, it can also suggest the presence of abnormalities such as left ventricular hypertrophy—thickening of the walls of the left ventricle—and CAD. A person with atrial fibrillation will not have an S_4. This is because S_4 is associated with atrial contraction. The atria don't contract when a person has atrial fibrillation.

Abnormal heart sounds like "murmurs" can indicate significant narrowing or regurgitation of heart valves or other problems. Certain types of heart problems are associated with certain kinds of heart murmurs. Based on the type of heart murmur you have, your doctor will decide if it needs to be checked out further. An echocardiogram is the standard test used to do this.

However, many murmurs aren't associated with any significant heart problems. Your doctor will decide whether a murmur is significant or not based on many factors. These include where the murmur is heard, how loud it is, whether it has a high or low pitch, the type of sound it produces such as harsh, "blowing," or "musical," and what part of systole or diastole it is heard in.

The loudness of a murmur is described using a scale ranging from 1 to 6. A grade 1 murmur is very faint. The classic medical joke is that a grade 1 murmur is one that's so soft nobody but a cardiologist can hear it. At the other end of the loudness scale, a grade 6 murmur can be heard even with the doctor's stethoscope lifted a little off the chest. Loud murmurs, like those that are grades 4 through 6, can be associated with a "thrill." This term means that your doctor can actually feel the vibrations from the murmur with the fingertips or the flat part of the hand placed on your chest. If your spouse feels a thrill when he or she puts a hand on your chest, that's a good thing. On the other hand, if your doctor feels a thrill after placing a hand on your chest, that's probably a bad thing.

Your doctor will also listen for several other types of heart sounds. These include the "clicks" normally heard with artificial, mechanical heart valves; one or more clicks heard in some people with mitral valve prolapse; the "opening snap" associated with mitral stenosis; and the scratchy sound of a "pericardial friction rub" that can be heard in people with pericarditis.

Following the history and physical examination, your doctor will decide whether to order more tests to see whether you have heart disease. The tests ordered usually include blood tests to screen for diabetes and high cholesterol. Tests to check for abnormal levels of minerals like sodium and potassium, kidney and liver disease, and blood counts to check for anemia and other problems will also typically be done. Thyroid function tests are done when a person is found to have atrial fibrillation or atrial flutter. This is because abnormally high thyroid function—hyperthyroidism—is a cause for these abnormal heart rhythms. Thyroid function tests are also checked when a person is discovered to have a significantly weakened left ventricle with no obvious cause, such as a known previous heart attack. Both excessively high or low thyroid function can cause the left ventricle to not work as well as it should.

An EKG and a chest X-ray will also usually be done. Both the EKG and chest X-ray may be normal even in patients with severe CAD or other heart problems. Nonetheless, they may show many other types of problems. For example, the EKG will detect abnormalities in the way the heart conducts electricity and arrhythmias like atrial fibrillation. A chest X-ray may show fluid in the lungs caused by heart failure.

Tests for Arrhythmias

Depending on what kind of heart problem your doctor thinks you may have, he or she may order some of the tests we've described previously, like an echocardiogram or a stress test. Other tests are used to check for intermittent problems with abnormal heart rhythms (arrhythmias). These tests are used in someone who is having episodes of frequent palpitations, has significant periods of lightheadedness, or has actually passed out. A "Holter monitor" is a small box with a recording device and tape cassette inside. A person typically carries the Holter monitor for about 24 hours. The Holter monitor is attached by wires to sticky patches on your chest and records the heart rhythm continuously.

While wearing the Holter monitor you record any symptoms you have, such as palpitations or lightheadedness, and the time the symptoms occurred in a small diary. Later a technologist scans the tape with all this information and your doctor gets a report of every single heartbeat you had. The report tells what your heart rhythm was doing when you felt any symptoms and even identifies abnormalities that occurred when you didn't feel anything, such as when you were asleep.

A limitation of the Holter monitor is that heart rhythm problems may be intermittent and unpredictable. While the Holter monitor tells exactly what's going on with your heart rhythm when it's attached to you and recording, it doesn't tell what happened the day before or the day after you used it. Any arrhythmia you had on the days you didn't have the Holter monitor on won't be detected.

An "event monitor" is a smaller box used to check for intermittent arrhythmias. Like a Holter monitor, it is attached to a person with wires connected to sticky patches on the chest. Unlike the Holter monitor, an event monitor is typically worn for weeks at a time and records the heart rhythm only when you or someone else pushes a button on it. If you feel palpitations or other symptoms you push this button to record your heart rhythm. This recording can be transmitted over the telephone to a monitoring center where it can be printed out. Your doctor later receives a report of what your heart rhythm was at the time you had your symptoms.

People with rare episodes of serious symptoms such as passing out can also use an "insertable loop recorder." This small device is similar to an event monitor but is implanted under the skin of the chest. When a person feels palpitations, lightheaded, or passes out, this individual or someone nearby activates the loop recorder wirelessly with a small handheld transmitter as soon as possible. Like an event monitor, the loop recorder then records the heart rhythm that occurred at that time. This recording is later retrieved from the loop recorder wirelessly using a radio transmitter/receiver device that "interrogates" the recorder. Some new loop recorders can even sense and record an arrhythmia automatically. A loop recorder can work for over a year inside the body and is eventually removed.

Cardiologists sometimes do more complicated tests to evaluate people who have episodes of passing out. A "tilt table test" involves placing the patient on a special table that tilts the person upright for a time. Normally, blood pressure drops only mildly and heart rate increases a little when a person goes into this position. However, people with "vasovagal syncope"—passing out due to an abnormal fall in heart rate or blood pressure, particularly under certain conditions such as standing, passing urine, getting blood drawn, etc.—are likely to have these abnormal changes occur during this test. They can then receive appropriate treatment.

A much more complicated test is an "electrophysiology study." This requires a cardiologist with specialized training—an "electrophysiologist"—to insert wires through a vein and sometimes an artery. These wires are then positioned inside the heart. The technique for inserting and positioning these wires is similar to the one we described for temporary transvenous pacemakers in Chapter 7. The wires are attached to an external recorder that measures the electrical impulses generated at different parts of the heart's conduction system. It can then tell if there are areas that don't conduct these impulses as well as they should. These wires can also stimulate the heart, like a pacemaker does. This stimulation is used to see if there are areas with abnormal conduction or if a person is at risk of having serious arrhythmias like ventricular tachycardia.

Magnetic Resonance Imaging and Computed Tomography
Besides all these standard tests we've described, two newer methods for detecting CAD and other heart problems are advancing rapidly. These are magnetic resonance imaging and computed tomography.

Magnetic resonance imaging (MRI) involves placing the person in a large magnet. Its powerful magnetic field produces different effects on the body's various tissues and organs. The MRI machine processes this information and produces very detailed images of these internal body parts. MRI is already an excellent tool for assessing blockages in other arteries of the body, such as the carotid arteries and the arteries that supply blood to the kidneys. It can also check for a dissection—a tear—or an aneurysm in the aorta and other blood vessels. A major advantage of MRI is that, unlike CT or other X-ray tests, it doesn't expose a person to radiation. Another advantage is that MRI does not require a person to receive an intravenous injection of the usual type of X-ray contrast (dye), which can cause allergic-type reactions and other side effects.

One disadvantage is that MRI can't typically be done in patients with a pacemaker or other metal in the body that could be affected by the magnetic field. However, new methods are now being developed to allow people with pacemakers to have MRI studies. The technologist or radiologist will go through a checklist with you prior to the MRI to see whether you can safely have the test. Also, some MRI machines require the patient to be placed in a smaller enclosure than others. About 15% of people may feel anxious and claustrophobic, unable to lie still long enough to get the test done. Some of them may be able to have the test if they are given medication to relax them.

MRI can also provide important information regarding abnormalities in the structure of the heart. MRI can also be used with stress testing in a way similar to an echocardiogram or a myocardial perfusion imaging study, as we discussed in Chapter 8. However, MRI's current ability to find blockages in the coronary arteries is limited by the heart being in constant motion and the relatively small size of the coronary vessels. Imagine trying to take a picture of someone who's jumping around while you're snapping the photo! With further improvements in these machines and scanning techniques, however, MRI will likely give sharp enough images of the coronary arteries to use it to screen for blockages. Stay tuned!

Computed tomography (CT) is a specialized form of X-ray machine that can, like MRI, be used to evaluate the aorta and other blood vessels. It can also be used to study the heart in several major ways. CT can detect the presence of increased amounts of calcium in the arteries of the heart, which is often, though not always, associated with blockage of those arteries. A person's "calcium score" tends to increase normally with age, with some older individuals having calcium in their arteries even without significant blockage. On the other hand, a calcium score that is high for a person's age could indicate the need for further testing for CAD, such as a stress test. Guidelines for dealing with these issues are now being developed.

Very advanced 64-slice CT scanners are also used to take pictures of the coronary arteries themselves. The "64-slice" part refers to the number of detectors the machine uses to obtain X-ray images of a selected area of the body. Roughly speaking, the higher the number of "slices" the faster these X-ray pictures can be taken and the sharper the pictures. As with MRI, movement of the heart during the test and the relatively small size of these vessels limited the quality of CT images in the past. However, unlike the current generation of MRI machines, the newer CT scanners are really ready for "prime time." Their images of the coronary arteries now rival those obtained with coronary angiography, the test that is our "gold standard" to check for CAD.

However, getting good CT pictures of the coronary arteries requires certain conditions. The patient must be able to hold his or her breath for about 10 seconds. The heart rate must be regular and slow enough—no faster than about 60 to 80 beats per minute—so that the heart isn't moving too much while the CT scan is taken. Slowing the heart rate often requires injecting a beta-blocker medication into a vein. The same type of contrast, X-ray dye, used for coronary angiography, with the same risks of using it we discussed previously, must also be injected into a vein. In addition, the CT scan also exposes the patient to a radiation dose that is about the same as doing the usual type of coronary angiogram. Coronary arteries with at least moderate calcification—a finding that increases the chance of having CAD but is often seen in elderly patients even without significant coronary blockages—cannot be adequately evaluated with the CT scan.

The current guidelines for using CT and MRI to evaluate the heart were published in the *Journal of the American College of Cardiology* in October 2006. A CT coronary angiogram can be used in certain patients with an "intermediate" risk of having CAD. A person with intermediate risk is considered to have anywhere between a 10% to 90% chance of having CAD based on age, gender, and presence of risk factors such as diabetes and high blood pressure. A CT coronary angiogram is appropriate if a person with intermediate risk for CAD either can't exercise well enough to do an exercise stress test, or has abnormalities on the EKG that prevent it from being used to tell if the heart isn't getting enough blood during a stress test.

A person with intermediate risk of CAD can also have a CT coronary angiogram under certain conditions if he or she has a long episode of chest pain. These conditions are that the person doesn't have EKG changes indicating the heart isn't getting enough blood, and the cardiac enzymes we discussed in

Chapter 7 don't show evidence of new damage to the heart. A CT coronary angiogram can also be used in a person who has a stress test whose results don't definitely tell whether significant CAD is likely to be present or not. Another indication for a CT coronary angiogram is to see if a person has a coronary artery that originates from an abnormal location—a "coronary anomaly."

An MRI of the heart can be used with a pharmacologic stress test (see Chapter 8) to assess suspected or known CAD. Like CT, MRI can also be used to see if a coronary anomaly is present. MRI is also helpful for assessing masses and suspected tumors within the heart, as well as evaluating complicated abnormalities of the heart and its major blood vessels due to congenital heart disease (heart problems present from birth—see Chapter 13).

Tests for Arterial Disease

Blockages in the carotid arteries can be detected using an ultrasound test. This test is similar to what's done with an echocardiogram. A transducer probe is placed over the carotid arteries. The ultrasound machine checks for blockage by taking pictures of the arteries and checking for abnormal blood flow within them.

MRI using a special type of contrast agent can also be used to check for blockages in the carotid arteries and other arteries of the brain. Doing MRI of the head at the same time can also check for evidence of an old stroke or other abnormalities within the brain. A CT scan of these arteries and of the head can also be used. However, it may not provide as much information as MRI does.

An ultrasound test can also be used to check for the presence of an abdominal aortic aneurysm (AAA).

This test is used when a mass with a strong and widened pulse is found in the middle of the abdomen. Even if they don't have this finding, men 60 years of age or older should have a screening ultrasound for AAA if they have a parent, brother, or sister who's had an AAA. An ultrasound test for AAA is also recommended for men between the ages of 65 and 75 who have ever smoked. MRI or CT may also be used to check for an AAA.

Blockages in the arteries to the legs can also be evaluated with ultrasound. An even simpler test to screen for blockages in these arteries is to check the "ankle-brachial index." This is the systolic blood pressure measured at the ankle divided by the systolic blood pressure measured in the arm on that same side of the body. This number is normally at least 1.0. A measurement of 0.9 or less suggests there is blockage somewhere in the arteries of the leg. MRI or, less commonly, CT can also be used to check for blockages in the arteries of the legs.

At times, a procedure similar to coronary angiography is used to check for blockages in the arteries to the brain, kidneys, legs, etc. Doing an "arteriogram" involves inserting a catheter into an artery in the arm or leg and threading it to the artery to be checked. As X-ray contrast is injected into the artery, a fluoroscope machine shows if there are any areas of narrowing. An arteriogram is usually done to see if blockages in the artery can be treated with angioplasty or are more severe and require surgery. The procedures used to treat blockages in these arteries are similar to the ones used to treat CAD we'll discuss in the next chapter. Certain medications, including aspirin and cilostazol (Pletal), can also be used to treat problems such as pain caused by blockages in the arteries of the legs.

Medications for Heart Disease
After reviewing the results of your heart tests, your doctor may decide to refer you to a cardiologist for further evaluation and treatment. For example, if your stress test shows you may have significant CAD, the cardiologist will decide whether you need to have a coronary angiogram to evaluate this. Both your doctor and the cardiologist may, in the meantime, prescribe medications for your heart problems.

Some types of medications we've discussed before can actually be used to treat more than one kind of heart problem. Beta-blockers are good for treating CAD, hypertension, and heart failure. They can decrease how often people with CAD get chest pain (angina) due to the heart not getting enough blood. Beta-blockers can slow down arrhythmias such as atrial fibrillation and flutter. This group of medications can prevent other kinds of arrhythmias, such as paroxysmal supraventricular tachycardia or premature ventricular contractions, from starting. Beta-blockers are also useful for less common heart problems, such as hypertrophic obstructive cardiomyopathy.

Angiotensin-converting enzyme (ACE) inhibitors and angiotensin receptor blockers are useful for treating hypertension, heart failure, and moderate to severe regurgitation of the mitral valve or aortic valve. These medications are also useful in many people with CAD, especially those with a recent heart attack, and people with reduced heart function from any cause. Both ACE inhibitors and angiotensin receptor blockers lower blood pressure but have little effect on the heart rate.

Both nitroglycerin and a similar type of medication, nitrates, can treat chest pain. However, they can also be useful for mildly lowering blood pressure and treating people with reduced heart function and heart failure.

Besides their value for treating CAD, the blood thinners aspirin and clopidogrel are also used in people with blockages in the carotid arteries to reduce risk of stroke. A medication similar to clopidogrel, ticlopidine, can also be used. However, it is more likely to cause certain serious side effects than clopidogrel, such as making the number of white blood cells in a person's blood decrease.

As we discussed in Chapter 6, atrial fibrillation and atrial flutter are arrhythmias that can increase a person's chance of having a stroke. Younger people with atrial fibrillation or flutter who aren't otherwise at increased risk of a stroke only need to take aspirin to reduce this risk. However, people at least 65 years old and those with hypertension, heart failure, or mitral stenosis should take a more powerful blood thinner, warfarin, to reduce this risk as much as possible. Warfarin is also used in people with artificial mechanical heart valves; those found to have blood clots in the heart or legs; and some people with blockages in the carotid arteries. Being a more powerful blood thinner than aspirin, the risk of bleeding is higher with warfarin. A blood test must be done at certain times to make sure a particular dose of warfarin is keeping the blood at the right level of "thinness." Sometimes warfarin and a low dose (81 mg) of aspirin are used together.

Calcium antagonists are a major class of heart medications we haven't discussed before because they have limited value in someone having a heart attack. However, they are very useful in people with hypertension and those with CAD who aren't having a heart attack. Diltiazem and verapamil are calcium antagonists that, like beta-blockers, slow the heart rate and lower blood pressure. They can be used to reduce heart rate in people with atrial fibrillation and flutter.

Several other calcium antagonists such as nifedipine, nicardipine, amlodipine, and felodipine also lower blood pressure. However, unlike diltiazem and verapamil, these calcium antagonists usually don't decrease a person's heart rate. Nifedipine and these similar calcium antagonists are more effective than diltiazem or verapamil for treating people with certain heart problems, such as severe mitral regurgitation or aortic regurgitation. Side effects from calcium antagonists are uncommon. Diltiazem and verapamil can cause fatigue, constipation, or stomach upset. Nifedipine, nicardipine, amlodipine, and felodipine are more likely than diltiazem and verapamil to cause leg swelling due to fluid retention.

Diuretics ("water pills") are used to treat excess fluid retention from any cause. People with heart failure in particular are susceptible to retaining fluid. Diuretics come in several different varieties. Low doses of "thiazide" diuretics, such as hydrochlorothiazide, are used to treat hypertension and mild fluid retention. Hydrochlorothiazide is often combined with another blood pressure-lowering medicine, such as an ACE inhibitor, in a single pill.

Spironolactone is another type of weak diuretic. It can actually improve survival in some people with severe heart failure. Amiloride is a weak diuretic that works differently from thiazide diuretics and spironolactone. Amiloride can be used to treat congestive heart failure or hypertension.

"Loop" diuretics like furosemide, bumetanide, and torsemide are more powerful than these other kinds. They can be given either in pill form or, especially in people with severe congestive heart failure, through a vein.

The major problem with most diuretics is that, besides their good effect of ridding the body of extra fluid, they can also deplete it of certain minerals such as potassium and magnesium. That is why people who take diuretics chronically are often prescribed potassium tablets—less commonly, magnesium pills too—to replace these minerals. Eating certain foods high in potassium such as bananas can also help. Spironolactone and amiloride are exceptions to this rule. Unlike other diuretics, these two medications can actually make potassium levels in the blood rise mildly.

Sometimes a diuretic may reduce the amount of fluid in the blood stream too much, causing dehydration and reduced kidney function. This can happen even when there might still be excess fluid and swelling in the legs. This can make it difficult to adjust the dose of the diuretic so that its good effects are maximized and its bad ones are minimized.

Digoxin is an old heart medication whose use was first formally described by Dr. William Withering way back in the late 1700s. It is one type of "digitalis"—a group of chemicals obtained from the leaves of the foxglove, a flowering plant whose technical name is *Digitalis*. Today, digoxin has been largely replaced by newer heart medications. However, it is still used occasionally for certain heart problems, either in a pill or intravenous form. Digoxin increases how forcefully the heart contracts and can be used to treat heart failure. It usually causes little or no change in blood pressure. Digoxin causes little change in heart rate in people who are in normal "sinus" rhythm. However, in those with atrial fibrillation or atrial flutter and a fast heart rate, digoxin can slow the heart rate back toward normal.

Digoxin's major limitation is that the difference between a dose that's helpful and one that's harmful is very small. The blood level of digoxin is measured to see if too much or not enough of it is getting into the bloodstream. A level that is too high can cause nausea and vomiting, fatigue, problems with vision, arrhythmias—and potentially, even death.

Ranolazine is a new heart medication for treating angina that was approved by the Food and Drug Administration in January 2006. It can be used if other medications such as beta-blockers or certain calcium antagonists haven't been effective enough or can't be given due to their side effects. Ranolazine usually causes little change in blood pressure or heart rate. Its potentially most serious side effect is that it might make a person more likely to have a serious, potentially life-threatening arrhythmia. Using ranolazine with certain other commonly used medicines, including several heart medications such as diltiazem or verapamil, could further increase the risk of having a serious arrhythmia.

We've already mentioned several medications such as lidocaine and amiodarone that are used to prevent and treat certain types of arrhythmias. Lidocaine is given intravenously and isn't effective if it is taken orally. However, several medications with effects similar to lidocaine, such as mexilitene and tocainide, can be given in the form of a pill. These two medications can be used to suppress serious arrhythmias originating in the ventricles, such as ventricular tachycardia. Possible side effects of mexilitene and tocainide include lightheadedness, nausea, tingling, and fatigue.

Flecainide and propafenone are similar medications used to treat arrhythmias occurring either in the atria, such as atrial fibrillation or atrial flutter, or in the ventricles. Their side effects include dizziness, headache, and nausea. They can mildly reduce heart function, which might cause heart failure in people whose heart is already weak. Flecainide and propafenone are used only very cautiously in people with CAD. This is because one large study showed flecainide and encainide, a similar medicine that's no longer available, actually increased the risk of dying in people who were otherwise doing well after a heart attack.

Sotalol is a beta-blocker with additional effects that suppress atrial and ventricular arrhythmias. Its side effects are the same as other beta-blockers. In certain people sotalol may even cause serious arrhythmias. It is usually started while a person is monitored in the hospital, where any new abnormalities on the EKG or occurrence of new arrhythmias can be caught as soon as possible.

Several old antiarrhythmic agents, such as quinidine and procainamide, are still available. Quinidine is typically given as a pill, while procainamide can be given either as a pill or intravenously. These two medications can be used to suppress arrhythmias originating in the atria or the ventricles. Quinidine and procainamide are not often used anymore due to their side effects and the availability of newer, more effective medications. However, they can be used if other antiarrhythmic agents don't work or aren't tolerated.

Finally, some older medications for treating hypertension are still occasionally used. One group includes clonidine and methyldopa. Their major side effects include fatigue, dry mouth, and drowsiness. Clonidine can be used either as a pill or as a long-acting patch.

Medicines like prazosin, doxazosin, and terazosin are now used less for treating hypertension than they are for a totally different problem—an enlarged prostate gland. These medications can cause lightheadedness and leg swelling. If one of these medicines is stopped for a few days and then restarted, blood pressure may fall too much when a person stands up—"orthostatic hypotension," to give this problem its technical name. This can make the person lightheaded or even pass out. To help avoid this, people taking prazosin, doxazosin, or terazosin for the first time ever, the first time at a higher dose, or the first time after they've stopped taking it for several days should take their medicine at bedtime. A person who is in bed and sleeping is less likely to have problems with blood pressure falling too much with these medicines than one who is standing up during the day. After one of these medicines is taken for a day or two, this problem with orthostatic hypotension is significantly less likely to occur.

Labetolol is a medicine that combines both the good and bad effects of a beta-blocker and medicines such as methyldopa. It can be taken as a pill to treat chronic hypertension. Labetolol can also be given intravenously to lower blood pressure more rapidly in a person with severe hypertension.

Minoxidil and hydralazine are medications that make arteries expand (dilate), thus lowering the blood pressure. Both can cause excessive fluid retention. While minoxidil and hydralazine are now only occasionally used to treat hypertension, each has found a place treating other problems. The combination of hydralazine and nitrates can be used to treat heart failure in people who can't tolerate either an ACE inhibitor or an angiotensin receptor blocker. One side effect of taking minoxidil as a pill is that it can make hair grow on unusual parts of the body. Used in a cream and rubbed on the scalp, however, this side effect is used to treat certain kinds of baldness.

The last major type of commonly used heart medication is cholesterol-lowering medicines. Cholesterol is measured in a blood test taken at least 10 to 12 hours after a person last ate anything. However, you can drink water and take your usual medications anytime before this test. A "fasting lipid profile" measures the total cholesterol, the triglycerides, and the high-density lipoprotein cholesterol—HDL, or "good" cholesterol. The low-density lipoprotein cholesterol—LDL, "bad" cholesterol —is usually not measured directly. Instead it is calculated in a simple formula using these other measurements. Take the total cholesterol, subtract the HDL value, then subtract one-fifth (20%) of the triglycerides—and the number you have left is the LDL. However, when the triglycerides are too high—more than 400 mg/dl—this formula can't be used. In that case, LDL needs to be measured directly in a separate blood test.

Generally speaking, the risk of CAD increases as the levels of triglycerides and LDL increase above normal and decreases as the HDL level rises. The current recommendations for cholesterol levels are strictest for people with known CAD. These same strict levels apply to individuals with an increased risk of having or developing CAD—diabetics and people with blockages in other arteries, especially in the legs.

Target values in these individuals are an HDL level more than 40 mg/dl; LDL at least below 100 mg/dl and preferably less than 70 mg/dl; and triglycerides less than 150 mg/dl.

The target levels for LDL in particular for people without CAD or these other problems are more complicated. Men 45 years old or older; women 55 years old or older; people who smoke, have hypertension, or an HDL less than 40 mg/dl; and those with a parent, brother, or sister who had CAD at an early age will have target LDL levels lower than those who don't. It is recommended that people with two or more of these risks factors try to lower their LDL with a low-cholesterol diet and exercise if LDL is 130 mg/dl or more. Using medications to lower it to below 130 mg/dl can also be considered, especially if the LDL is greater than 160 mg/dl. For people with one or none of these risk factors, an LDL of 160 mg/dl or more should also be treated with diet and exercise. Medications to lower cholesterol can also be considered in these individuals, especially if the LDL is greater than 190 mg/dl.

Lowering the amount of cholesterol and fats in the diet, eating more fiber (such as oat bran), losing weight if you're overweight, and exercising usually lower LDL by an average of about 5 to 10%. However, due to the inefficient way their bodies handle cholesterol, some people may notice no change in their LDL even when they do all these things. On the other hand, other people may see their LDL fall up to about 25% with exercise and eating a healthy diet.

If the targets for cholesterol can't be reached by these simple measures alone, a large number of cholesterol lowering medications can be used. The most helpful class of these medicines is the "statins" or, much more formally, HMG-CoA reductase inhibitors. These include lovastatin, simvastatin, atorvastatin, pravastatin, and rosuvastatin. They work primarily by lowering LDL. However, they may also mildly increase HDL and decrease triglycerides. Some, like atrovastatin and rosuvastatin, are more potent than others. Several, like lovastatin and simvastatin, are more effective when taken around bedtime than in the morning.

Statins have been shown to be particularly helpful in people with CAD and those with blockages in the arteries of the neck and legs. They not only lower LDL but also have other beneficial effects that reduce risk of heart attack, stroke, and death. They can reduce the chance a blockage in an artery will get worse and may even make the blockage smaller. Statins also make it less likely that a blood clot will form on a blockage.

Although most people have no problems taking them, statins can occasionally cause muscle soreness or pain, belly cramping, headache, or constipation. Rarely, statins can cause muscle damage or make blood tests for your liver function abnormal. However, these bad effects go away when the medicine is stopped. Your doctor will periodically check your liver function blood tests when you are taking a statin. If you develop significant muscle pain or other evidence of possible muscle damage, a blood test to check for this will also be done.

Several other, less potent medications are also used specifically to lower LDL. Ezetimibe works well either by itself or in combination with a statin. Uncommon side effects include diarrhea and joint pains.

Cholestyramine and colestipol are taken as powders mixed with water and juice. Colesevelam, a similar medication, can be taken as a tablet. These three medications are collectively known as "bile acid sequestrants." They lower LDL and may increase HDL. Triglyceride levels remain about the same or may even rise. The main limitation of these medications is that each of them can cause bloating and constipation.

Gemfibrozil and fenofibrate are members of a class called fibrates. They primarily lower triglycerides. However, fibrates can also mildly reduce LDL and mildly increase HDL. This class of medicines has been found to reduce risk of heart attacks. Side effects include stomach upset, belly pain, and nausea. Fibrates may also very mildly increase the risk of developing gallstones.

Niacin (nicotinic acid) is the cholesterol-lowering medication that usually raises HDL levels the most. It also mildly reduces LDL and triglycerides. Unfortunately, many people develop side effects with niacin. These side effects are not life-threatening but may be uncomfortable enough to limit how much niacin they can take. The most common side effects with niacin are flushing, sweating, and itching. Starting a low dose of niacin and gradually increasing the dose, or using an extended-release form of it, can significantly reduce problems with these side effects. Taking niacin before bedtime and about 30 minutes after taking a dose of aspirin (81 to 325 mg) can also be helpful.

Cardiology in the Future

As you see, the number of tests and medications available to treat a person with a heart attack or other heart problem has increased tremendously since the man in 1965 we've talked about previously had his chest pain. Coronary angioplasty and echocardiograms, calcium channel blockers and statins—so much of what we take for granted today wasn't even dreamed of back then.

It's difficult to imagine how cardiology will be practiced in another forty years or so. New blood tests are being evaluated for their usefulness in identifying people at risk of developing CAD. Elevated blood levels of C-reactive protein and homocysteine are reported to increase a person's risk of developing CAD. However, the best ways to treat people with elevated blood levels of these substances are still being determined. There has also been research suggesting that atherosclerosis, including CAD, may be at least partly due to certain infections and might even be treated with antibiotics!

New technologies, such as positron-emission tomography (PET), have also been developed to evaluate certain kinds of heart problems. While the standard myocardial perfusion imaging tests we described in Chapter 8 are done with thallium-201 and technetium-99m, PET uses other types of "low-level" (mildly) radioactive substances to scan the heart. Some of these "radiotracers" used with PET can evaluate blood flow to the heart as a part of a pharmacologic stress test to see if a person has CAD. PET can also be used to see if an area of the heart is permanently damaged or if it is "hibernating"—not working as well as it should due to limited blood getting to it, but capable of working better if the blood supply is restored.

Eventually, techniques using stem cells—that is, cells able to transform into heart muscle or other types of cells—and genetic engineering may be used to grow back blood vessels or heart muscle in a damaged heart. For example, recent studies have suggested that a person with extensive heart damage can be treated by injecting stem cells from the person's own bone marrow into heart muscle or into a coronary artery supplying blood to the damaged area of the heart. It is thought that some of these bone marrow cells may help produce new heart muscle cells and blood vessels to improve heart function. While preliminary results are encouraging, with some patients showing improvement in their heart function, research is still being done to see how useful this technique will be.

Eventually, genetic engineering might even be used to grow a "replacement" heart itself! However, for now this possibility is still science fiction.

In the next chapter we'll move on to another topic—the procedures and types of surgery we have to treat heart disease.

Chapter 9 Summary

- ♥ Initial evaluation for possible heart disease includes a history and physical examination, blood tests, and simple tests such as an EKG and chest X-ray.

- ♥ Magnetic resonance imaging (MRI) and computed tomography (CT) are used to assess for abnormalities in the structure of the heart and major blood vessels.

- ♥ Computed tomography can be used to check for calcification and blockages in the coronary arteries.

- ♥ Many effective medications are now available to treat coronary artery disease, high blood pressure, heart failure, arrhythmias, and abnormal cholesterol levels.

♥ New tests such as positron-emission tomography (PET) and treatments such as stem cell therapy are still being developed to evaluate and treat heart disease.

Chapter 10: Mending a Broken Heart
Procedures and Operations for the Heart and Blood Vessels

Chapter Preview:
Coronary Angioplasty
    Basic technique for coronary angioplasty
    Atherectomy and other procedures
Restenosis After Coronary Angioplasty
    Medications used to prevent restenosis
    Coronary stents
    Brachytherapy
Coronary Artery Bypass Surgery
    Indications for coronary artery bypass surgery
    Techniques for coronary artery bypass surgery
Transmyocardial Laser Revascularization
    Indications and methods
Enhanced External Counterpulsation
    Indications and procedure
Artificial Heart Valves
    Types of artificial heart valves
    Anticoagulation with warfarin
    Valvotomy for mitral stenosis
Surgery for Aortic Dissection and Aortic Aneurysms
    Grafts and stent-grafts
Surgery for Carotid and Other Arterial Disease
    Angioplasty, endarterectomy, and grafts
Surgery for Congenital Heart Disease
    Procedures and surgery
Cardiac Transplantation
    History and success rate of cardiac transplantation
    Late complications of cardiac transplantation
Mechanical Hearts
    Total artificial hearts
    Ventricular assist devices

Pacemakers and Implantable Cardioverter-Defibrillators
  Permanent pacemakers
  "Twiddler's syndrome"
  Implantable cardioverter-defibrillators
  Ablation and maze procedures

UNLIKE JUST ABOUT everything else, it takes more than duct tape to repair a broken heart or damaged blood vessel. In this chapter we'll discuss the tools, techniques, and hardware cardiologists and cardiovascular surgeons use to help fix these vital parts of your body.

Coronary Angioplasty

When Henry did his cardiology training in the early 1980s, a new procedure was just starting to become available. Now "percutaneous transluminal coronary angioplasty"—PTCA, or coronary angioplasty for short—is a mainstay of care for coronary artery disease (CAD). Over nine hundred thousand people in the United States alone had this procedure in 2003—and the number of people having it is increasing.

As we described in Chapter 7, coronary angioplasty is the preferred way to treat one major type of heart attack—"ST-elevation myocardial infarction." Coronary angioplasty is also the usual procedure for treating significant blockages when they are present in only one or two coronary arteries. Blockages more than 70% are most suitable for the procedure. However, coronary blockages between 50% and 70% may also sometimes benefit from coronary angioplasty. The initial success rate of coronary angioplasty is good and the risk of serious complications such as heart attack or death is low.

Chapter 10: Mending a Broken Heart

The basic technique for doing coronary angioplasty hasn't changed significantly over the years. Like coronary angiography, it involves inserting a long thin tube called a catheter into an artery and threading it back to the heart. Unlike the catheter used for angiography, the angioplasty catheter has an inflatable balloon at the end. A long guide wire that fits through the catheter is advanced until it goes through the opening of a partially blocked artery. The catheter itself is then moved forward, using the guide wire as a "track" as to where it should go. The tip of the catheter is pushed into the area of blockage.

The balloon at the end of the catheter is then inflated under high pressure. This widens the opening inside the narrowed coronary artery. The balloon flattens the area of the blockage and partially tears the blood vessel wall. It also "cracks" any part of the blockage that's hard and rock-like from the presence of calcium. Ultimately, more blood can then get to the area of heart muscle beyond the blockage. This helps relieve chest pain or other problems caused by the heart not getting enough blood.

In a way, the cardiologist doing coronary angioplasty is acting like a high-tech "plumber." The pipes in your home can get clogged with minerals such as calcium from hard water going through them. They may need to be unclogged by one of the snake-like tools your plumber uses to clear them. Roughly speaking, the cardiologist does something similar to blocked arteries. The major difference is that the cardiologist's bill is even higher than the plumber's.

The balloon catheter is by far the most common device used to open clogged arteries. However, over the past two decades other techniques have been developed to reduce blockage in the coronary arteries. One is a "cutting balloon" catheter. This is a special type of balloon catheter with three or four fixed blades at the end. These blades cut into the blockage when the balloon is inflated. This can make it easier to compress the blockage and increase blood flow in the artery.

Several types of more complicated catheters are used to perform an "atherectomy." This procedure uses a catheter to directly cut or grind away an area of blockage. "Directional coronary atherectomy" uses a catheter with a metal cylinder at its end. The cylinder contains an electric cutting unit with a small blade. This cylinder is partially open on its side. Wires connect this cutting device to an electric motor outside the patient. The cardiologist positions the tip of the catheter inside a coronary blockage, then turns the motor on. The cutting blade then spins at about two thousand rotations per minute, shaving off atherosclerotic plaque through the opening in the side of the cylinder.

A hollow cone at the tip of the catheter collects the shaved off material from the plaque. Without this cone, debris from the plaque would travel "downstream" through the artery. This material would eventually block off the artery as it became smaller. This would damage heart muscle since blood couldn't reach it through the blocked artery.

A fancier version of this atherectomy device uses a pair of rotating blades. It also connects the catheter to a vacuum system on the outside of the patient. As the blockage in a coronary artery is sliced away, debris is sucked back through the catheter to keep it from causing harm. Other types of catheters are also used to help prevent this "showering" of removed plaque. One type uses a second balloon that's partially inflated beyond the blockage. Another uses a small filter at the end. All of these catheters are designed to collect debris and remove it from the body.

"Rotational coronary atherectomy" works in a similar way. Instead of a blade, it uses a rough burr at the end of a catheter to grind a coronary blockage away. This burr is coated with tiny chips of diamond and spins at about one hundred sixty thousand rotations per minute. It is most effective for treating blockages that are very hard and calcified. In this case the cardiologist has something in common with your dentist, who uses a similar but much larger version of this tool to smooth out rough areas on a new filling.

There are even catheters that shoot a laser beam at a coronary blockage. No, don't think of flashing crimson and emerald death rays like in *Star Wars*. First, the light from the laser is in the ultraviolet or infrared range—you couldn't see it if the catheter were "turned on" outside the patient. Second, the laser beam produces only a little heat and doesn't work primarily by "zapping" the plaque. Instead its light energy produces "shock waves" that break up the plaque. It also causes a chemical reaction in the blockage that helps the body itself to remove the plaque.

Sometimes, to help decide which of these procedures is best for a particular person, the cardiologist can take a more direct look at blockages in the coronary arteries. As we discussed in an earlier chapter, coronary angiography uses X-ray contrast to check for areas of blockage in the coronary arteries. However, the contrast only outlines the inside of the artery. It only indirectly identifies blockages by showing areas that are "pinched off" compared to other, presumably more normal parts of the artery that show more blood getting through them.

Sometimes the coronary artery may look more "normal" than it actually is due to the area of blockage not being seen at the best angle, or if the artery has significant blockage throughout its length. "Intravascular ultrasonography" is one method used to check on how severe a blockage actually is. A special catheter with ultrasound transducers at its tip is inserted into a coronary artery. This catheter takes black-and-white pictures of the inside of the artery and any blockage within it using the same basic techniques as the echocardiograms we described in Chapter 8.

"Coronary angioscopy" uses a special catheter with a fiber optic system inside it that can display an actual color picture of the inside of a coronary artery on a television monitor. This technique lets the cardiologist see exactly what an area of blockage or a blood clot inside a coronary artery looks like.

A major limitation to using either intravascular ultrasonography or angioscopy to evaluate the coronary arteries is that the special catheters used for these procedures can't look inside arteries smaller than the catheter itself is. Likewise, the catheter can't see beyond a blockage in a coronary artery that has an opening too small for the catheter to get through. A cardiologist must also have special training and experience to do intravascular ultrasonography or coronary angioscopy.

Restenosis After Coronary Angioplasty
Atherectomy and laser catheters do a better job than balloon catheters in only a small percentage of patients who have certain types of complicated blockages. The two major advancements in the past quarter century for improving long-term results from coronary

angioplasty are actually rather low-tech. Both deal with what happens *after* the angioplasty is done.

A serious problem during the early years of balloon angioplasty was the high rate of "restenosis." This means that a coronary blockage (stenosis) treated with angioplasty became worse again weeks or months after it was successfully opened up. The blockage might even become worse than it was before the angioplasty! Restenosis occurred in about a third of people treated with angioplasty, usually within the first six to nine months after the procedure.

Restenosis is caused mainly by blood clots and scar tissue forming where coronary angioplasty damaged the inner lining of the artery. Research showed that restenosis was more likely to occur with certain complicated types of blockages and in people with certain medical problems such as diabetes. In those situations, other treatments such as coronary artery bypass surgery (see below) were thought to be possibly better than balloon angioplasty.

New blood-thinning medications and placing a tiny metal mesh called a stent in an artery after angioplasty have dramatically reduced the rate of restenosis. Before, during, and after angioplasty a patient can be treated with several "old" blood thinners such as aspirin and heparin. New blood-thining medications such as abciximab, eptifibatide, and bivalirudin are given intravenously only around the time of the procedure. Clopidogrel is a new oral medicine that is also begun around the time of angioplasty. It is taken with aspirin for a period of time ranging from one month to a year (typically three to six months) after a stent is placed. Clopidogrel is often then stopped, but aspirin is continued indefinitely.

A stent is a tubular metal mesh positioned in the part of the blocked coronary artery opened up by the balloon catheter. It is placed on the tip of a special balloon catheter. When the balloon is inflated in the artery, the stent expands and acts as a support to keep the artery from partially collapsing. Stents have generally been made of stainless steel. Newer ones use different metal alloys, such as cobalt chromium.

These original "bare metal" stents significantly reduce the risk of restenosis compared to using angioplasty alone. However, further improvements have occurred in the past several years with the introduction of "drug-eluting" stents. These stents have a thin coating containing a medication that comes into contact with the wall of the artery. The medication reduces inflammation and scar tissue formation. Two antibiotics, sirolimus and paclitaxel, are used in these drug-eluting stents to reduce the risk of restenosis.

The combined use of all these medications and different varieties of stents has significantly reduced the overall risk of restenosis after angioplasty. The average risk of restenosis in the first six months after angioplasty is now as low as 10% or less. Research is currently being done to determine whether or not one type of drug-eluting stent is better than another, and to define the indications for using a bare metal stent versus a drug-eluting stent in particular patients. One concern based on recent data is that drug-eluting stents may have a higher rate of forming blood clots in the coronary artery treated long after they are placed than bare metal stents do. As more research is done, the recommendations for what types of stents should be used and how long clopidogrel should be continued after stent placement may change. Cardiologists performing angioplasties will follow the latest recommendations for placing stents and using medications after the procedure.

One final technique—"brachytherapy"—can be used in the relatively uncommon situation when a patient develops restenosis within the stent itself. A mildly radioactive material is inserted into the area of the stent by a special catheter. The low-level radiation applied there reduces the risk of scar tissue forming and closing the stent again.

Coronary Artery Bypass Surgery
Coronary artery bypass graft surgery (CABG) is the other major procedure besides coronary angioplasty used to treat coronary disease. The first CABG was done in 1964. It was the only major procedure used to treat coronary disease until coronary angioplasty became widely available in the early 1980s.

About 500,000 CABG operations were done in the United States in 2003. The number done each year has actually decreased over the past decade. As coronary angioplasty techniques have advanced, many people who would have had CABG in years past now have the less complicated coronary angioplasty. CABG is a major operation and is done by cardiovascular surgeons. In contrast, specially trained "interventional" cardiologists perform coronary angioplasty. As we've talked about earlier in this chapter, coronary angioplasty requires only needle puncture of an artery and not surgically cutting open the chest.

CABG is most useful for people with severe, extensive CAD. This includes those with significant blockages in all three coronary arteries or in the left main coronary artery. Like coronary angioplasty, CABG is very effective for relieving angina. CABG also significantly reduces the future risk of death compared to treatment with medicine alone in some people. This includes people with disease of the left main coronary artery and those with both severely reduced left ventricular function and three-vessel coronary disease.

In the "classic" form of CABG, after the patient is given a general anesthetic and is asleep, the surgeon performs a "sternotomy." A small electric saw with a circular blade is used to cut through the sternum (breast bone), exposing the heart. Medications are used to stop the heart. The patient's circulation is maintained with a cardiopulmonary bypass (heart-lung) machine. Tubes inserted into a large artery and a large vein carry blood to and from the machine. There carbon dioxide and other waste products are removed and blood supplied with oxygen is returned to the body. Basically, the heart-lung machine gives the heart a rest, so the surgeon doesn't have to work on a "beating target."

The surgeon makes an incision on one or both legs to remove part of a vein that's located there—the saphenous vein. One end of a section of this vein is sewn into the aorta, not far above the aortic valve. The other end of the vein is sewn into a diseased coronary artery beyond where the blockage is located. Thus, the vein acts as a pipe that "bypasses" the blockage. Blood flows through this "vein graft" between the aorta and the coronary artery. Other sections of the vein are used to bypass blockages in other coronary arteries. These vein grafts help supply the heart with as much blood as possible.

Unfortunately, veins weren't designed to carry the high-pressure blood from the aorta they are called on to do after CABG. Although they usually hold up well for a long time, each year there's a small chance one of these vein grafts will deteriorate or clot off. By 10 years after CABG, the chance of any one of these vein grafts being open and working is about 50% or less.

For this reason, whenever possible surgeons use one of the two internal mammary arteries as a bypass graft. The internal mammary artery is a branch of one of the major arteries in the chest, the subclavian artery. Since its near end is already connected to an artery, the surgeon only has to separate the internal mammary artery out from its surrounding tissue. The far end of the internal mammary artery is then cut and sewn into the diseased coronary artery beyond its area of blockage. By far the most common procedure is to use the left internal mammary artery to supply blood to a diseased left anterior descending artery.

The major advantage of using the internal mammary artery instead of a vein is that the artery is already accustomed to carrying high-pressure blood. It is far less likely than a vein to deteriorate and clot off over time. The chance of an internal mammary artery graft being open after 10 years is over 90%. This is significantly higher than the 50% or so chance of a vein graft remaining open.

One downside of using an internal mammary artery graft is that it takes the surgeon more time to do this type of graft than a vein graft. This makes the operation longer, and so an internal mammary artery graft may not be the best choice for emergency surgery. Also, a person has only two internal mammary arteries. If, as is often the case, there are blockages in multiple coronary arteries, some of them will usually need to be bypassed with leg veins. Other arteries, such as the radial artery—the one used to check for a pulse in your wrist—or the right gastroepiploic artery, located in the upper abdomen, can also be used for a bypass graft.

Needless to say, opening a person's chest and using a heart-lung machine is major surgery. In recent years, techniques for so-called "minimally invasive" bypass surgery to reduce the overall risks of surgery have been developed. One of them requires a sternotomy, but it does not use a heart-lung machine—"off-pump" bypass surgery.

Another approach involves making an incision in the left side of the chest instead of going through the sternum and avoids use of the heart-lung machine. This operation has a lower rate of complications and shorter recovery time than doing a sternotomy. However, since only the "front" of the heart can generally be reached with this technique, it's usually limited to patients who need only an internal mammary graft to the left anterior descending artery. Blockages in other arteries usually can't be treated with this method.

"Port-access" bypass surgery requires a heart-lung machine but not a sternotomy. Tubes placed in the front of the left chest allow the surgeon enough access to the heart to place grafts, especially when an endoscope—a probe that lets the surgeon directly see the heart—is used.

Overall, about 80% of patients requiring CABG surgery still need the usual type of operation with a sternotomy and heart-lung machine. However, a growing number of people are candidates for these newer techniques.

Transmyocardial Laser Revascularization

Transmyocardial laser revascularization (TMLR) is used to treat patients with CAD too severe to be adequately helped by coronary angioplasty or CABG. A cardiovascular surgeon typically performs TMLR by making an incision in the chest to see the heart. The surgeon places a laser probe on the area of the left ventricle that is not getting enough blood. The thin beam of light from the laser is used to burn many narrow channels through the wall of the left ventricle to its cavity. This allows blood from inside the left ventricle to directly flow into the heart muscle. The tiny holes produced by the laser beam on the outside of the left ventricle seal themselves off by clotting and eventually forming scar tissue.

The reasons why patients do better after TMLR are still debated. Besides potentially helping a person because blood is now getting into heart muscle from the left ventricular cavity, the tiny holes made in the left ventricle's wall may also stimulate production of very small blood vessels within it. These very small blood vessels may also help supply the heart with blood and improve both chest pain and heart function in a person with severe CAD.

TMLR can be done by itself, with the surgeon making an incision in the left side of the chest to see the heart directly. The surgeon may also make a smaller incision and use a special tube-like device called a thoracoscope to look at the heart when TMLR is performed. A person having CABG through a sternotomy may have TMLR done at the same time if it is thought CABG alone will not be enough to improve blood supply to all areas of the heart.

Enhanced External Counterpulsation
Enhanced external counterpulsation (EECP) is another, much simpler method used to treat chest pain caused by severe CAD. EECP does not involve taking medications or surgery. Inflatable cuffs similar to blood pressure cuffs are wrapped around a person's legs at the level of the calves, lower thigh, and upper thigh. A

special device inflates and deflates these cuffs at specific times as the heart beats.

During diastole, when the left ventricle is not contracting, the cuffs inflate. This sends blood from the veins back to the heart, which increases how forcefully the left ventricle will contract with its next beat during systole. Diastolic blood pressure also increases when these cuffs inflate, which helps get more blood through the coronary arteries to the heart. This may also stimulate very small blood vessels ("collaterals") in the heart to provide more blood to heart muscle supplied by coronary arteries with blockages. The cuffs deflate during systole. This reduces the pressure the left ventricle has to contract against and gets more blood to the rest of the body.

EECP is given as series of treatments. Each treatment is typically given an hour at a time. Each of these hour treatments can be given 5 days per week for 7 weeks, for a total of 35 hours. EECP may help reduce the number of medications people with CAD need to treat their chest pain, decrease how often they get chest pain, and increase the amount of exercise they need to do before they develop chest pain.

EECP can be an effective addition to medical therapy for patients with chest pain whose CAD is so severe that it cannot be treated adequately with coronary angioplasty or CABG. Patient with certain medical problems cannot have EECP. These include patients with severe heart valve disease, uncontrolled hypertension, very rapid heart rate, severe congestive heart failure, and significant peripheral arterial disease involving the iliac or femoral arteries supplying blood to the legs.

Artificial Heart Valves

When they aren't bypassing coronary arteries, cardiovascular surgeons keep busy repairing or replacing heart valves and diseased aortas, as well as treating patients with peripheral arterial disease.

Artificial (prosthetic) heart valves have been used since the early 1960s. They come in two major varieties—mechanical valves, made completely of artificial materials like metal and plastic, and tissue (bioprosthetic) valves, which are partly made of animal or human tissue.

The earliest successful mechanical valve was the Starr-Edwards valve. This valve consists of a metal ring that is covered by a cloth made of plastic fibers coated with Teflon. A metal cage with a plastic ball inside is attached to the bottom of the ring. After a diseased mitral or aortic valve is removed at surgery, the ring part of this artificial valve is sewn into the spot where the person's "original" valve used to be. The ball and cage part is positioned so that it is "downstream," beyond where a normal valve would be. For example, with a mitral valve the ring is sewn into the opening between the left atrium and the left ventricle, while the ball and cage part is actually in the left ventricle itself.

As blood flows through the Starr-Edwards valve the ball moves to the far end of the cage, allowing blood to get through. When blood stops going through it the ball moves to the near end of the cage and prevents blood from leaking back to where it shouldn't go. An artificial mitral valve "closes" when the left ventricle is contracting (systole). An artificial aortic valve closes when the left ventricle isn't contracting (diastole).

The vast majority of mechanical valves used today are "tilting disc" valves, such as the St. Jude valve. Instead of a ball and cage to regulate blood flow, this type of valve use a ring with one or two metal discs inside it that pivot on tiny rods. The discs tilt and allow blood to flow through the ring when it's supposed to, then tilt back and cover the opening in the ring so blood can't leak back where it came from. In a way it acts like a much smaller and more sophisticated version of a toilet bowl lid.

These mechanical valves have proven very durable. Some Starr-Edwards valves are still working four decades after they were implanted. However, the major disadvantage of mechanical heart valves is that, having only artificial parts, they have a significant risk of blood clots forming on them. As a rule, artificial mitral valves are more likely to form blood clots than aortic valves.

People with a mechanical heart valve need to take an oral blood "thinner" for the rest of their lives to reduce this risk of a blood clot forming on the valve. Warfarin (Coumadin), taken as a pill, is the anticoagulant used to do this. This medication makes blood less likely to "coagulate" (clot) by interfering with a chemical inside your body, vitamin K. Your body uses vitamin K to help make certain substances—"clotting factors"—needed to make blood clot.

Taking warfarin at the right dose decreases the risk of blood clots forming to about a third of what it would be without this medication. However, if the dose used is too potent and the blood becomes too "thin," warfarin can cause bleeding in various parts of the body. On the other hand, if the dose of warfarin is too small the blood isn't "thin" enough, and the risk of blood clots increases.

The right dose of warfarin varies from person to person. Even in the same person it can be hard to maintain the right level of blood "thinness." One reason for this is that many other medications a person may also be taking can change how effective warfarin is. Some of these other medications interfere with warfarin, so more warfarin is needed to get the blood "thin" enough. Others make warfarin more potent, so less warfarin is needed. Even eating certain foods containing vitamin K, such as green leafy vegetables, reduces the effects of warfarin. And sometimes the effectiveness of a particular dose of warfarin changes for no obvious reason at all.

A specific blood test, the INR, is used to see whether a person's dose of warfarin is right or not. It often needs to be done every week or two until the best warfarin dose is found, then usually every four to six weeks or so after that. The usual target for the INR in people with a mechanical heart valve is 2.5 to 3.5.

Tissue ("bioprosthetic") valves have been used since the mid 1960s. Most use a pig's valve that's been treated with certain chemicals. This valve is then placed in a cloth-covered ring with metal supports. Besides these "porcine" valves, the tissue (pericardium) surrounding a cow's heart can also be used to form the leaflets for a valve. Less commonly, valves from human cadavers are used.

The major advantage of a tissue valve is that it is far less likely to develop blood clots than a mechanical valve. Except for the first few months after surgery, a person with a tissue valve does not routinely need to take warfarin. The major disadvantage of a tissue valve is that it isn't nearly as durable as a mechanical valve. Over time, tissue valves deteriorate and may need to be replaced again. As a rule, this happens more rapidly in younger people than in older ones. Tissue valves are generally not used in anyone less than 35 to 40 years old. They are used only in special circumstances in younger people, such as those who are at very high risk of bleeding with warfarin.

Deterioration of a tissue valve occurs much more slowly when the valve is placed after age 65. Elderly people are more likely to die from other causes before their tissue valve needs to be replaced. Older people also generally have a higher risk of bleeding from the warfarin needed with a mechanical valve. For these reasons, a tissue valve is the preferred type of artificial valve used in the elderly.

Some young people who need replacement of their aortic valve—for example, due to severe aortic stenosis—can be treated with the "Ross procedure." In this operation, the person's own normal pulmonic valve is removed and used to replace the diseased aortic valve. A treated aortic or pulmonic valve taken from a human cadaver is then inserted where the original pulmonic valve was removed. A major advantage of the Ross procedure is that the person's own pulmonic valve, used to replace a diseased aortic valve, is less likely to deteriorate than an artificial valve made from animal tissue. Patients having the Ross procedure also do not need to take warfarin.

Both mechanical and tissue valves share two other limitations. These valves typically have a smaller opening than a normal heart valve, which at least mildly limits blood flow through them. Any type of artificial valve is also associated with a small risk of becoming infected—"infective endocarditis," which we discussed in Chapter 6. Infected artificial valves often need to be replaced.

If a leaking heart valve is not too severely damaged, the surgeon may be able to repair it instead of replacing it. This is most commonly done with the mitral valve, but it can also be done with the other valves. The surgeon may cut and place sutures in one or both leaflets of the mitral valve to tighten it. An artificial ring (annuloplasty ring) can be sewn around the valve's outer rim to help keep it tight.

As we discussed in Chapter 6, mitral stenosis can cause serious symptoms in both young and old people. If mitral stenosis is severe enough, especially if the person has significant symptoms despite treatment with medications, several types of procedures can be done. A less severely diseased mitral valve can be treated with a "balloon valvotomy." This procedure is usually done by a cardiologist rather than by a surgeon. Like angioplasty, it uses a catheter with an inflatable balloon on the end. One technique inserts the catheter into a vein in the leg and advances the catheter to the right atrium. From there, the catheter passes through the interatrial septum—usually by a needle puncture—to the left atrium. The tip of the catheter is guided into the stenotic (narrowed) mitral valve from its "upper" side. The balloon is then inflated and "widens" the narrowed mitral valve.

The balloon catheter can also be passed to the mitral valve from the opposite direction. In this technique, the catheter is inserted into an arm or leg artery and threaded into the left ventricle. From there its tip is inserted into the "lower" side of the mitral valve before inflating the balloon.

More severely diseased mitral valves may be treated best with a surgical valvotomy. The heart surgeon can do a "closed" valvotomy. This does not require placing the person on a heart-lung machine. A "dilator" is placed in the left ventricle and used to widen the mitral valve without the surgeon seeing the valve itself. For the most part, however, this procedure has been replaced by balloon valvotomy, which is generally more effective and carries lower overall risk.

An "open" valvotomy does require a heart-lung machine. The chest is actually opened so the surgeon can see the mitral valve. This operation carries somewhat more immediate risk for the person, but it does the most extensive repair on the diseased mitral valve. The valve is widened by slicing away the scar tissue and hard lumps of rock-like calcium that form on it. Open valvotomy also lets the surgeon remove a small part of the left atrium—the left atrial appendage—where blood clots tend to form. This helps decrease the long-term risk of stroke. Also, if the surgeon sees that the valve is too damaged to repair, it can be replaced then and there.

All these procedures can make the mitral valve work better, but they don't make it normal again. Over time, the mitral valve will worsen. However, valvotomy procedures can delay the time before the valve needs to be replaced by about a decade or more.

While a balloon valvotomy can help many people with severe mitral stenosis, its value for treating severe aortic stenosis is much more limited. It can be used in some children and young adults for treating severe aortic stenosis present from birth—"congenital" aortic stenosis. The leaflets of the valve in these individuals are usually relatively thin. They can often be successfully "stretched" with the inflatable balloon to allow more blood to get through the aortic valve.

However, severe aortic stenosis is far more common in older adults. In them, the stenotic aortic valve is usually hard and calcified. This makes it more difficult to open up the valve with the balloon and to keep it open afterward. Up to about 75% of adults with severe "calcific" aortic stenosis will have some initial improvement in the amount of narrowing of the valve following balloon valvotomy. However, in about half of them the valve will narrow down again to a significant degree within the next six months. In one recent study, only 18% of adults who had this procedure were alive and without symptoms two years later. As a rule, balloon valvotomy is used only as a temporary treatment in symptomatic adults with severe calcific aortic stenosis who are too ill to have an aortic valve replacement.

Surgery for Aortic Dissection and Aortic Aneurysms
Aortic surgery is needed when the inner lining of part of the aorta tears. This may be due to high blood pressure or other causes. This "aortic dissection" may even cause rupture and bleeding from the aorta and is life-threatening. While aortic dissection is most common in the elderly, it can happen in younger people too. John Ritter, the well-known actor, died of an aortic dissection at age 54. Depending on how severe and extensive the dissection is, the surgeon may be able to open the aorta and repair the area where it tore. If the damage is too severe, the diseased part of the aorta may need to be replaced with an artificial tube (graft).

The aorta can also start to bulge, forming an aneurysm. Although this can happen to the part of the aorta in the chest, it's more common in the belly (abdomen). The major risk of an "abdominal aortic aneurysm" is that, after it reaches a certain size—a little over two inches in diameter—it has a high risk of rupturing. The standard operation to prevent this requires opening the aneurysm through an incision in the belly. An artificial graft is then placed inside the aorta before closing it again.

Recently, special grafts have been developed that can be placed in the aorta through the femoral artery—the same artery in the groin used for coronary angiography. This avoids surgery on the belly itself. This "stent-graft" is somewhat similar to the stents used to treat coronary arteries, but it is much larger. Unfortunately, many people aren't candidates for this particular procedure due to the size and extent of their aneurysm or other technical factors.

Surgery for Carotid and Other Arterial Disease
Several procedures can be done to treat blockages in arteries besides the coronary arteries, particularly the arteries that supply blood to the legs. Specially-trained cardiologists, radiologists (physicians trained to interpret and perform tests using X-rays), and surgeons can do angioplasty of blockages in these arteries and place stents in them. The technique used is similar to balloon angioplasty of coronary arteries. Many of the other methods used to treat CAD we talked about earlier in this chapter, such as laser systems, can be used to treat blockages in the arteries of the legs and elsewhere.

A surgeon can also treat blockages in some of these other arteries, particularly the carotid arteries, with an "endarterectomy." This involves opening the diseased artery and directly removing atherosclerotic plaque from it. Surgeons can also use a vein or artificial graft to bypass a blocked artery, particularly an artery in the leg. The principle behind this procedure is similar to what's done during a CABG, with the vein or graft "bypassing" the area of blockage to supply blood to the diseased artery.

Surgery for Congenital Heart Disease
Cardiothoracic surgeons occasionally do procedures to correct or improve serious heart defects that are

present at birth. The most serious of these "congenital" heart defects can involve very complicated plumbing changes to make the heart and its major arteries work better.

"Simpler" heart defects might not need to be worked on until children are older. They might not even be detected until adulthood. For example, the surgeon can open the heart and place a small patch to cover an abnormal opening between the right atrium and left atrium—an "atrial septal defect"—or the two ventricles—a "ventricular septal defect." A small blood vessel that causes an abnormal connection between the aorta and pulmonary artery—a "patent ductus arteriosus" —can be tied off through a chest incision.

Repairing these types of heart defects used to be the sole domain of the surgeon. Now cardiologists can treat some of them without surgery. Some atrial septal defects can be plugged with a small occluding device placed by a catheter. A different kind of plug placed using a special catheter can also block off the abnormal blood vessel present with a patent ductus arteriosus.

The most severe congenital heart defects require cardiac surgery that can be very complicated. Babies and young children may have congenital heart defects so severe they need surgery as soon as possible to treat their symptoms or even to keep them alive. Before operations to treat them were devised, many of these unfortunate children with severe congenital heart defects did not survive to adulthood. Now, with special surgery, their quality of life and chances of living longer are significantly better.

Because there are so many kinds of these severe congenital heart defects, with so many different kinds of operations used, we'll hold off describing them in

Cardiac Transplantation

detail here. We will describe some of them in Chapter 13.

Cardiac Transplantation

Cardiovascular surgeons still have a monopoly on the most radical type of heart procedure—cardiac transplantation. The first successful human heart transplant was done in 1967 by Dr. Christian Barnard. Henry remembers attending a talk by him years ago. Dr. Barnard described some of the exotic surgical methods that were later tried but turned out to be of limited value. These included replacing the diseased heart with a baboon heart or adding a second "piggyback" heart—either baboon or human—to the diseased heart without removing it.

The vast majority of heart transplants involve a basic "take the bad part out and put the new one in" principle familiar to any auto mechanic. Considering the seriousness of the operation, the risk of heart transplant surgery itself is relatively small. Rejection of the "foreign" or donated heart by the patient's body turned out to be the major problem in the first few years the operation was done. Early medications used to suppress this reaction were not very effective and lowered the body's resistance to infection. The net effect was that, between 1967 and 1971, the chance of being alive a year after a heart transplant was only 15%—better than 0%, but with great room for improvement.

Survival after heart transplantation has improved dramatically since then. This is due to new methods for early diagnosis of rejection of the new heart and due to better ways to prevent and treat rejection. "Endomyocardial biopsy" is a procedure done by cardiologists in which a catheter-like device is inserted through a vein and positioned in the right ventricle. Tiny movable metal jaws at the tip of the device "bite" away a sliver of the heart muscle, which is then removed. A pathologist reviews the sample under a microscope for the telltale signs of rejection. If rejection is present, special medications can be used to treat it. Some of the medications used to prevent and treat rejection include cyclosporine, tacrolimus, corticosteroids, antithymocyte globulin, and special kinds of antibodies.

Several other problems can occur years after heart transplantation. Long-term use of medications used to suppress rejection increases the risk of developing a life-threatening infection and cancer. However, development of a particularly nasty variety of CAD is the major problem that limits long-term survival. The "usual" form of CAD generally involves isolated blockages ranging from mild to severe. However, the coronary disease associated with heart transplantation typically is present throughout the whole length of the coronary artery. It progresses more rapidly and involves more arteries than usual. This type of coronary disease also commonly responds poorly to the medications and procedures, like angioplasty, normally used to treat CAD.

Mechanical Hearts

The total artificial hearts developed so far have allowed a small number of people to live days to months without their original heart. These artificial hearts have included the Jarvik-7, as well as the newer AbioCor model that's placed entirely in a person's chest. The major problems with these devices have included blood clots forming in them, causing strokes or other problems, and infections. This is an area where more research is clearly needed. By the way, did you know that the person who patented the first artificial heart was Paul Winchell, the great ventriloquist of Jerry Mahoney and Knucklehead Smiff fame? Clearly, *he* was no dummy. (Sorry about that. With apologies to Dr. McCoy from *Star Trek*, Henry says, "I'm a cardiologist, not a comedian!")

A "ventricular assist device"—a mechanical pump used to help rather than replace a weakened heart—can be very helpful in some patients. This device can be used to help the left ventricle, the right ventricle, or both. A ventricular assist device requires placing tubes into appropriate areas of the heart and its blood vessels. These tubes are then connected to a pump that is totally outside the body or, with the newest models, can actually be placed inside the body. For example, to support a weak left ventricle, a tube placed in the left atrium sends blood to the pump, which then propels it back into the body via a tube inserted into the aorta.

A ventricular assist device can be used as a temporary treatment to "bridge" people to heart transplantation, supporting them until a donor heart is available. In some individuals who are not candidates for heart transplantation, the device can even be used permanently. A ventricular assist device can also be used until a person's heart recovers from a temporary problem. For example, myocarditis (inflammation of the heart muscle) can severely weaken the heart. However, heart function may improve significantly over the course of days to weeks. The ventricular assist device is used to support the person's heart until this improvement (hopefully) happens.

Pacemakers and Implantable Cardioverter-Defibrillators

There are several procedures used to treat arrhythmias that are done by both cardiologists and surgeons with specialized training. Pacemakers are electronic devices that, in their typical form, are used to treat abnormally slow heart rates. If a person's own heart rate is too slow to pump blood to the brain and rest of the body, blood pressure falls and they may feel lightheaded, pass out—or die.

In Chapter 7 we discussed how a "temporary transvenous pacemaker" is used to treat a person with a heart attack whose heart rate has fallen dangerously low. An individual whose heart rate doesn't recover after a heart attack may need to have a pacemaker permanently implanted inside the body. People with a variety of other problems with the heart's electrical system can also have intermittent or chronic problems with dangerously low heart rates and require a permanent pacemaker.

A permanent pacemaker replaces the heart's own malfunctioning electrical system. It contains a "pulse generator" that produces electrical impulses. One or two leads—thin, plastic-coated wires—are attached to the pacemaker. A battery within the pacemaker powers this system. The first pacemaker systems were introduced in the late 1950s and were very simple, bulky devices. They were worn outside the body, with their wires inserted through the chest directly into the wall of the left ventricle. You set the rate you wanted the heart to beat, and that was it.

Modern pacemakers resemble these earliest models as much as the room-size vacuum tube computers of the 1950s resemble a modern laptop. New pacemakers are, in fact, miniature computers. These devices are small enough to place under the skin, beneath a collarbone. The doctor doing the procedure—a specially-trained cardiologist or a cardiovascular surgeon—numbs the skin with an injected anesthetic, makes an incision (cut), and places the pacemaker into a pocket under the skin. A lead is inserted into a nearby vein and threaded to the end of the right ventricle. The other end of the lead is attached to the pacemaker. Another lead is usually placed in the right atrium—a "dual-chamber pacemaker." At the end of the procedure, the skin over the pacemaker is sewn up.

The pacemaker generates electrical impulses that go through the lead(s) and directly stimulate the appropriate heart chamber to contract. Dual-chamber pacemakers, with leads in both the right atrium and right ventricle, help the heart pump blood more efficiently than if only the right ventricle is paced.

The pacemaker can be programmed to beat at different rates and with different types and timings of electrical signals. This is done using a small radio transmitter/receiver on the outside of the body that is placed near the pacemaker. Modern pacemakers can also be "rate-adaptive." This means the pacemaker can automatically speed up the heart rate when it's needed, such as when a person is exercising (that includes having sex).

The batteries used in earlier pacemakers might last only a few years or less. Modern pacemaker batteries may function well for up to about 10 years. Pacemakers are checked periodically to make sure they are operating correctly. The battery inside the pacemaker is monitored to see if it is becoming weak. The type of battery used is designed to gradually lose its power over time and not fail suddenly. When the battery does reach a certain level of depletion, the entire pacemaker is replaced with a new one, with a new pulse generator and battery. The old pacemaker lead inside the heart is usually not replaced but simply connected to the new pacemaker.

The chance of having a serious problem after a pacemaker is placed, such as infection or serious bleeding, is low. Fortunately, with modern pacemakers failure of the pacemaker generator itself is uncommon. Occasionally, a lead can move enough so that it doesn't stimulate the heart muscle as well as it should. The lead's connection at the pacemaker might also come loose or part of the wire system inside the lead can break.

One reason why a pacemaker might not work right is "twiddler's syndrome." A person with a pacemaker may "twiddle" with it—perhaps inadvertently, perhaps even deliberately moving it around with his or her fingers. This can make the pacemaker rotate in the pocket and pull the pacemaker lead(s) out of the heart. This prevents the pacemaker from doing its job of stimulating the heart. Since the pacemaker doesn't know the lead isn't where it belongs, it keeps on sending electrical impulses into the lead. Depending on what part of the chest its tip is now close to, the lead might now stimulate a nearby muscle or nerve. This can make the arm or a chest muscle on the same side of the body where the pacemaker is located "twitch" or jump. It can also make the person feel pulsations in the belly (abdomen). The lesson here is, the one thing neither you nor your spouse should "twiddle" with is your pacemaker!

A pacemaker is an electrical device. A strong magnet or electrical field might cause "electromagnetic interference," or EMI, and prevent a pacemaker from working correctly. Fortunately, modern pacemakers can be safely used around most common electronic and electrical devices, including personal computers, microwave ovens, and vacuum cleaners, as long as these machines are used properly. However, some devices, such as arc welding equipment, airport security systems, and even certain types of cell phones might potentially cause problems with the pacemaker. Ask your doctor for details about what devices are and aren't safe with your particular pacemaker and heart problem.

Pacemakers are also occasionally used for reasons other than to treat abnormally slow heart rhythms. For example, certain people with severely weakened hearts may benefit from "biventricular pacing." This is also known as "cardiac resynchronization therapy." A pacemaker with two leads is used to stimulate both the right and left ventricle with just the right timing so they can work most efficiently. A third lead is also often placed in the right atrium with this therapy.

An "implantable cardioverter-defibrillator" (ICD) is a device that resembles a pacemaker. However, while a pacemaker is used to treat abnormally slow heart rhythms, an ICD treats dangerously fast heart rhythms like ventricular tachycardia or ventricular fibrillation. Like a pacemaker, an ICD is implanted beneath the collarbone, with a lead placed in the right ventricle. If a serious, potentially life-threatening fast heart rhythm like ventricular tachycardia occurs, the device senses it. The ICD then shocks the heart through that lead to restore normal rhythm.

For some types of abnormally fast heart rhythms, instead of shocking the heart the ICD can perform "antitachycardia pacing." This means the ICD fires a short burst of fast electrical impulses that stimulate the heart the same way a pacemaker does. These electrical impulses interrupt the abnormal fast heart rhythm and make it go away. The ICD even has a built-in memory, recording what the heart rhythm was when it shocked or stimulated the heart. This information can then be transmitted to an external device that can produce an EKG strip.

An ICD and a pacemaker can be combined in a single device. It is used in people who have both abnormally fast and slow heart rhythms. A device that is both an ICD and a pacemaker may have leads in both the right atrium and right ventricle. The most advanced ICDs can be used for biventricular pacing, as well as for treating both abnormally slow and fast heart rhythms.

ICDs are used in people who have survived a life-threatening episode of ventricular tachycardia or had ventricular fibrillation and are considered to be at significant risk of having one of these arrhythmias again. A person who has ventricular tachycardia or fibrillation at the time of a heart attack may or may not need to have an ICD. If the heart attack causes only mild heart damage or blood supply can be restored to enough of the heart by coronary angioplasty or CABG, an ICD might not be needed. However, people with moderate or severe heart damage may need to have an ICD implanted because they are at significant risk of eventually having another life-threatening episode of ventricular tachycardia or ventricular fibrillation. An ICD is also implanted in people who have not yet had life-threatening ventricular tachycardia or ventricular fibrillation but have a heart problem that puts them at high risk of someday having one of these potentially fatal arrhythmias.

Specially-trained cardiologists can perform "radio frequency (RF) ablation." This procedure "burns away" areas on the inner wall of heart chambers or other parts of the heart that cause abnormal conduction of electrical impulses. This abnormal conduction can produce a variety of arrhythmias. These arrhythmias include atrial fibrillation, atrial flutter, the most common types of paroxysmal supraventricular tachycardia, and ventricular tachycardia. A special catheter is inserted into a vein, usually in the leg but sometimes in the neck or beneath the collarbone. The catheter is then advanced to the heart. The area of abnormal conduction is then "ablated"—burned away—by the heat produced by radio waves generated at the tip of the catheter. They heat up the abnormal tissue to around 130 degrees Fahrenheit. This makes the tissue no longer able to conduct electricity.

Cardiovascular surgeons can also perform a "maze procedure" during heart surgery to treat atrial fibrillation. Several techniques are used for this. One involves making a series of shallow incisions with a scalpel in the inner lining of an atrium. These cuts are then sewn together to interrupt the abnormal electrical activity that causes atrial fibrillation. Another technique uses an electric cauterizing device instead to make these "cuts" in the atrium. There is also a variation of the maze procedure that requires only a small incision in the chest rather than major heart surgery. It uses a special probe that freezes areas of heart tissue to destroy its ability to conduct arrhythmias.

In this chapter, we've described a mind-boggling variety of heart procedures and operations. In the next one we'll talk about how they affect having sex.

Chapter 10 Summary

♥ Coronary angioplasty, atherectomy, and similar procedures use special catheters to treat coronary artery disease without surgery.

♥ Coronary artery bypass graft surgery (CABG) is an operation used to treat severe and extensive coronary artery disease.

♥ Transmyocardial laser revascularization and enhanced external counterpulsation (EECP) are procedures used to treat coronary artery disease too severe to be treated by coronary angioplasty and coronary artery bypass graft surgery alone.

♥ Artificial heart valves and procedures such as valvotomy are used to treat severe disease of the heart valves, particularly the mitral and aortic valves.

♥ Permanent pacemakers are used to treat serious slow heart rhythms. Implantable cardioverter-defibrillators are used to treat life-threatening fast heart rhythms.

Chapter 11: Sex After Surgery
From the Operating Room to the Bedroom

Chapter Preview:
Sex After Coronary Angiography
  Risk of bleeding after angiography
Sex After a Pacemaker
  Pacemaker and implantable cardioverter-defibrillator function
Sex After Heart Surgery
  Wound healing after heart surgery
  Cardiac rehabilitation programs and exercise

HEART DISEASE CAN limit a person's ability to have sex both physically and psychologically. The heart rate and blood pressure changes that normally occur with intercourse and the amount of energy needed to do it are modest. However, they can still be too much in people with moderate to severe heart disease. Intercourse can indeed cause angina and, though rare, myocardial infarction (heart attack) in people with coronary artery disease (CAD). Those with cardiomyopathies, severe valve disease, and abnormal heart rhythms can also find themselves unable to "keep up" with sex. They may become too short of breath or lightheaded to do it. Even just the fear of developing these symptoms during intimacy can be a major "turn off" for both partners. Although the risk is actually very low, the image of your loved one dying during sex is not a pretty one.

Treatment with medicines alone may not be enough to reduce these risks. As we'll see in the next chapter, some heart medicines may themselves have side effects that worsen bedroom performance. In many people, coronary angioplasty and bypass surgery can substantially improve their symptoms and return them to a safe sex life. In others, having valve surgery, getting a pacemaker, or other procedures can do the same thing.

Well, after the cardiologist or surgeon has finished working on your heart, how long should you wait before you can have sex again? We'll go into much more detail about when people with heart disease can safely have sex in the next chapter. Here we'll confine ourselves to discussing the limitations these specific heart procedures and operations themselves cause. In general, any restrictions or delays after having one of these procedures are not usually due to the heart itself—after all, the heart has been "repaired." Instead, any restrictions are related mainly to recuperating from the procedure itself.

Sex After Coronary Angiography
For the first few days after a coronary angioplasty or even a plain coronary angiogram, if the test was done in the usual way through an artery in the groin, moving the leg too much could cause bleeding or bruising in or near the groin. It's best to avoid activities that cause too much bending of the leg or putting pressure on it. While your doctor will likely tell you about not lifting anything heavy or driving for at least a few days, vigorous sexual activity with lots of motion and rolling around also falls into this category. If the area in the groin where your doctor punctured the artery is looking fine after several days to a week following the procedure, the risk of having bleeding from the puncture site during sex is most likely low.

Sex After a Pacemaker

Recovery time after placement of a pacemaker or implantable cardioverter-defibrillator (ICD) is usually short. The arm on the side where the device is placed is usually kept in a sling for about 24 hours after the procedure. After that, if the pocket where the pacemaker or ICD is placed isn't causing you any pain and the wound appears to be healing well, you may be able to resume sex as soon as about a week after the procedure. Of course, you should also check with your doctor first to make sure there are no other heart-related or other reasons to delay having sex besides having the new pacemaker or ICD.

Even if you're super unlucky and your new ICD fires during intercourse itself, the shock itself isn't dangerous to you or your partner—although it probably will spoil the mood of the moment. In fact, if the ICD weren't there, the serious abnormal heart rhythm it treated might indeed have led to death for you and a very bad memory for your partner.

One potential problem with older pacemakers is that they may be set to pace at only a single, pre-programmed rate. If your own heart rate can't increase during sex, and the pacemaker is still firing away at a rate of (say) 70 beats per minute when the body really needs a heart rate of 130 beats per minute, you may have shortness of breath or other symptoms. This isn't a problem, however, with other types of pacemakers, especially the newer rate-adaptive pacemakers. Check with your doctor to see if your particular pacemaker and heart rhythm problem lets the heart rate increase when it's needed.

Sex After Heart Surgery

Big operations, such as having the usual type of coronary artery bypass graft surgery (CABG) or a valve replacement, need longer recuperation times. For the first few days after the operation, pain from the surgery, nausea, lingering effects of the anesthetic, weakness from not being able to move around or getting any solid food, and so on make getting up to go to the bathroom—much less having sex—physically difficult. Under these circumstances, unless your sex drive is as powerful as a volcano, having sex will be really low on your priority list right after the operation.

By the time you're ready to go home from the hospital, however, you may well have recuperated enough to wonder when you can have sex again. Once again, if your doctor tells you the surgery went well, your heart usually won't be the limiting factor. Besides feeling well enough to "do it," the major limitation will be making sure you don't undo all the fancy sewing work the surgeon did to stitch you back together again.

The incisions on your leg where the surgeon removed part of your saphenous vein for a CABG can be quite long. These incisions have stitches that need to be kept clean and secure until the wounds have healed enough that they can be safely removed or, in some cases, absorbed by the body. You'd probably prefer to avoid calling your cardiovascular surgeon's office to confess you ripped open a wound by practicing exotic positions from the *Kama Sutra* too early after surgery. The rate of healing in these leg wounds varies a great deal from person to person. As a general rule, it's best to avoid disturbing these wounds until your surgeon makes sure they're healing well at your first office visit after the operation. This is usually about three or four weeks after the surgery.

The other vulnerable part of your body after most types of CABG and heart valve surgery is your breastbone (sternum). After the surgeon has cut through it, the sternum is now a broken bone held together, not with a cast, but with wire sutures beneath the skin. Like all broken bones, the sternum will take months—perhaps up to a year—to heal completely. The basic recommendation for deciding when it has healed enough to have sex is, "If it hurts when you do it, don't do it!" It typically takes about a month for a sternotomy wound to feel good enough to try sex in any position that puts significant strain on the sternum.

Even if your sternotomy wound doesn't hurt, it's prudent to avoid putting too much stress on the sternum. It's possible for those wire sutures to break or for the two parts of the bone to separate, especially during the first few months after surgery. We've seen it happen, and it was very painful for the patients. Being gentle, letting your partner assume the superior position, or using a side-by-side position during intercourse may reduce strain on the sternum. When any leg or other wounds have healed after his heart surgery, a man can also use a kneeling or standing rear-entry position with his wife. However, a rear-entry position is not a good idea if he's at risk of becoming lightheaded or passing out. This might be due to blood pressure dropping too low or, less commonly, an abnormally slow or fast heart rhythm occurring. This is a question that you need to ask your doctor about.

Sometimes it can take weeks or even months for a person to recuperate enough after heart surgery to have sex. Your muscles become "deconditioned"—work less efficiently—very quickly after surgery. This also happens with any illness that severely limits your activity for even a short time. It takes much longer to build your stamina back up than it does to lose it.

Participating in a cardiac rehabilitation program can help speed recovery after heart surgery or a heart attack. These programs help you gradually build up strength with various forms of moderate exercise, such as walking on a treadmill or pedaling a stationary bicycle. Your heart rate and blood pressure can be monitored to make sure you can exercise safely. Even doing a simple walking program on your own can be helpful. Regular periods of moderate exercise make your muscles work more efficiently. This means the heart has to work less to supply your muscles with blood and oxygen. You benefit by being physically able to do activities that require greater levels of energy—like sex. We'll discuss how much and how often to exercise in Chapter 15.

Loss of libido (sexual desire), anxiety, and depression are common after a heart attack or major heart surgery. They may, in fact, be far out of proportion to the actual physical effects of the heart problem or surgery. If this occurs, talk with your doctor about ways to deal with these psychological issues. Support from a spouse, participation in a cardiac rehabilitation program and, if needed, small doses of certain medications to relieve anxiety or depression can all be helpful.

As we've already mentioned, after heart procedures and surgery are done, the heart usually isn't the limiting factor in resuming sexual activity. However, there are exceptions to this rule. Sometimes neither the cardiologist nor the surgeon can treat every significant blockage in people with very extensive CAD. There may still be areas of the heart not getting enough blood, limiting what a person can do. Also, if your heart muscle was very weak before surgery, it may not recover completely. This is most likely to occur when the heart has been damaged and scarred by prior heart attacks.

An area of the heart may not contract strongly because it isn't getting enough blood through a partially blocked coronary artery. This "hibernating" heart muscle hasn't been permanently damaged. It will eventually improve its function and contract harder after it gets more blood following coronary angioplasty or CABG. Similarly, when a person has a heart attack, part of the heart may not get blood long enough to be "stunned," but not damaged. A stunned area of the heart may temporarily not contract normally even when its blood supply is improved, such as with coronary angioplasty. In fact, it may take weeks or months after angioplasty or CABG for hibernating or stunned heart muscle to recover and work better.

Until your heart recovers enough, your doctor may need to give you temporary restrictions on activity. These restrictions may include sexual activity. If there's a question about what level of activity you can safely do, your doctor may have you perform an exercise stress test. If it shows you can safely do at least a moderate level of exertion (more on this in the next chapter), sex may be OK. If in doubt, ask your doctor.

People having heart transplants have one specific problem. The transplanted heart is "denervated"—that is, its nerve supply has been interrupted by being removed and placed in another body. This means that the usual nerve impulses that would tell it to beat faster or harder in response to stress, exercise—and sex—aren't there anymore. The heart rate and amount of blood pumped from the heart with each beat may increase more slowly than normal. They may fall short of what's needed for a particular level of exercise, leading to shortness of breath and fatigue. Fortunately these limitations usually aren't serious enough to prevent someone with a heart transplant from being able to perform the moderate levels of activity needed for sex. However, you may be more comfortable if your partner does most of the muscular exertion.

The procedures and surgery we've described in this book help people with heart disease live longer and be more active. Part of their improved quality of life includes being able to have sex safely. In the next chapter we'll describe how some medications can help the heart but interfere with sex. We'll also tell how to deal with this problem.

Summary of Chapter 11

♥ Sex can usually be resumed within several days to a week after a coronary angiogram.

♥ Sex can usually be resumed about a week after a pacemaker or implantable cardioverter-defibrillator is placed if a person's wound is protected and the heart is doing well.

♥ Sex can usually be resumed about four weeks after heart surgery if a person's wounds have healed sufficiently and the heart is doing well.

♥ It may take weeks or months for a person's heart function and ability to exercise to improve as much as possible after heart surgery.

♥ A cardiac rehabilitation program or other exercise program can improve a person's ability to perform activities, including sex, after a heart attack or heart surgery.

Chapter 12: Pills and Penises
Medicines and Sexual Dysfunction in Men

Chapter Preview:
Erectile Dysfunction
    Definition
    Male sexual function and age
    Some causes of erectile dysfunction
Beta-Blockers and Sexual Dysfunction
    Risk of erectile dysfunction with beta-blockers
    Alternatives to beta-blockers
Other Heart Medications and Sexual Dysfunction
    Heart medications associated with sexual dysfunction
    Heart medications not associated with sexual dysfunction
Medications Used to Treat Sexual Dysfunction
    Viagra and similar medications
    Precautions for using Viagra and similar medications
Other Treatments for Sexual Dysfunction
    Other medications for treating erectile dysfunction
    Vacuum devices
    Penile implants
Heart Disease and Sexual Dysfunction
    Erectile dysfunction as an indicator of possible heart disease
    Erectile dysfunction and vascular disease
Evaluating the Safety of Sexual Activity
    Effects of sex on heart rate and blood pressure
    Level of exertion needed for sex
Assessing the Risk of Sex with Heart Disease
    Safety of sex with different types and severity of heart disease
    Heart tests used to evaluate safety of having sex
    Reducing risk to the heart during sex

As we discussed in earlier chapters, many new medications have been introduced to help people with heart disease. These medications reduce risk of heart attacks, stroke, and death. They improve quality of life by allowing people to be more active without having shortness of breath, chest pains, and other symptoms limiting what they can do.

Yet as wonderful as these new medications are, none are without side effects. When Henry prescribes a new medication, he tells his patient why he's giving it and what its most common and serious side effects are. One of the side effects he mentions is the possibility that a particular medication can cause problems with having sex.

Erectile Dysfunction
Many medications used to treat heart disease and other medical problems can cause erectile dysfunction (ED). ED refers to a man's inability to have or sustain an erection sufficient to complete sexual intercourse. Although healthy men can continue to have sex throughout their lives, some mild changes occur normally as they get older. Compared to younger men, older ones tend to achieve either partial or complete erections more slowly and may have less intense orgasms with fewer contractions. After intercourse it may take the older man's penis longer to "recover" before he can have another erection. During intercourse, however, he may be able to delay ejaculation longer than he could when he was younger. This latter change is perhaps a positive one from his wife's point of view.

It is normal for a man to have an occasional episode of ED. This can occur due to fatigue or psychological factors such as stress, anxiety, depression, guilt, or problems of any kind between his wife and him. It is abnormal for it to be a recurrent problem, to last more than several months or, worst of all, be present all the time (impotence). One way to see if a problem with ED has a significant psychological component is to see if a man can achieve erections by self-stimulation or if he has erections during sleep. The latter can be confirmed by the presence of an erection when he wakes up or by an episode of "nocturnal emission"—the technical name for a "wet dream."

ED can also be evaluated by placing a thin perforated tape around the penis (not *too* tightly!) at bedtime. The tape is checked in the morning to see if the penis broke it by becoming expanded and erect during the night. At a higher level of technology, "nocturnal penile tumescence testing" can also be done to check for erections during sleep. It uses a recording device to obtain more sophisticated and complete measurements of the number and quality of nighttime erections.

In otherwise healthy men, alcohol, tobacco, and medications like some antihistamines, narcotic painkillers, and sedatives can contribute to ED. Commonly used antidepressants such as tricyclic antidepressants or selective serotonin reuptake inhibitors (like fluoxetine or paroxetine) can also produce ED. Unfortunately, many of the medications used to treat heart problems also cause ED.

Beta-blockers and Sexual Dysfunction
It's ironic that one of our most useful classes of heart medications is also the one most associated with sexual dysfunction. Beta-blockers are useful for treating coronary artery disease (CAD), heart failure, hypertension, and abnormal heart rhythms (arrhythmias). However, despite their many beneficial

effects, beta-blockers can also decrease desire to have sex and cause ED. How beta-blockers do this is uncertain. It's thought beta-blockers may work directly on the brain to reduce libido. They may also reduce blood flow to the penis. There doesn't seem to be a significant difference between older beta-blockers, like propranolol, and newer ones, like metoprolol or atenolol, in causing these problems.

Beta-blockers reduce risk of death in people with weakened heart function, such as when heart muscle is damaged with a heart attack. However, sexually active men with damaged hearts may be reluctant to take beta-blockers due to their risk of causing sexual dysfunction. Without too much exaggeration, these men may see it as a choice between living longer or keeping life worth living.

However, recent studies have suggested that the risk of ED in men taking beta-blockers may be lower than once thought. The overall risk may be in the range of about 2%—a very low risk compared to the known benefits of these medications. In fact, the risk of developing ED in men taking beta-blockers may be more psychological than physical. In a study published in the *European Heart Journal* in 2003, a group of men without ED who were recently diagnosed as having hypertension or chest pain (angina) were all given the same dose of atenolol, one of the newer beta-blockers. One-third of them were not told what medication they were taking. Another third were told the name of the medication but not told it could have sexual side effects. The other third were told both the name of the medication and that it could cause sexual dysfunction.

After three months of treatment, only 3.1% of the men who weren't told what medication they were taking reported having ED. However, ED occurred in

15.6% of the second group of men, who knew they were taking a beta-blocker but weren't told it might cause sexual dysfunction. A whopping 31.2% of the men who knew both the name of the medication and its potential sexual side effects developed ED.

These results should not be taken as suggesting that physicians shouldn't tell their patients of a medication's potential side effects. That would be very questionable from an ethical standpoint. Besides, a patient can easily learn about any side effects from the package insert included with the medication, a friendly question posed to a local pharmacist, or an Internet search. Rather, it shows that sometimes knowledge of a side effect can lead to a "self-fulfilling prophecy." This might be especially the case with ED, which is so dependent on whether a man is anxious, depressed, or just worried about sexual performance after being told he has cardiovascular disease.

Men with diabetes or blockages in the arteries supplying blood to the penis may be more likely to develop ED with beta-blockers. Even in men without such problems, beta-blockers can cause ED independent of any psychological effects. If you're the one it happens to, then for *you* the risk is 100%. Knowing that most men don't get this side effect is no consolation at all—quite the contrary! In that case, the choices include decreasing the dose of the beta-blocker or trying an alternative heart medication that is less likely to cause ED.

Fortunately, for at least some cardiac problems there are good medications available that have similar benefits to beta-blockers but have rarely been associated with ED. Calcium channel blockers are, like beta-blockers, useful for treating high blood pressure and angina. Some, like diltiazem and verapamil, have effects similar to beta-blockers in reducing blood pressure and slowing heart rate. They are particularly useful in people with abnormally fast heart rhythms, such as atrial fibrillation, atrial flutter, or paroxysmal supraventricular tachycardia. Like beta-blockers, they can also be used in patients with hypertrophic obstructive cardiomyopathy.

Other calcium channel blockers, like nifedipine, felodipine, or amlodipine, are different from beta-blockers in that they have little effect on heart rate but are of similar value in lowering blood pressure. Calcium channel blockers are actually better than beta-blockers for the small group of patients whose chest pains are due primarily to their coronary arteries going into spasm and reducing blood flow to the heart.

However, in many cardiac patients beta-blockers are clearly superior to calcium antagonists. Diltiazem only very mildly decreases risk of death in one type of heart attack and only then when the overall function of the left ventricle is normal or near normal. When left ventricular function is moderately or severely decreased in these patients, however, diltiazem can actually increase the risk of dying. Conversely, beta-blockers, even in very low doses, may significantly improve survival in patients with heart attacks or other types of heart damage, especially if their overall left ventricular function is at least mildly reduced.

Verapamil and diltiazem can potentially worsen heart failure in patients with moderately to severely decreased heart function due to causes other than a heart attack. Other calcium antagonists, such as felodipine and amlodipine, are not generally used to treat heart failure. However, these calcium antagonists can be used cautiously to treat problems that could cause heart failure, such as severe mitral regurgitation or aortic regurgitation.

Henry's male patients with heart disease are prompt to tell him if they feel more short of breath or tired after he starts them on a beta-blocker. However, it's a different story when that same medication or others we'll discuss later cause bedroom problems. A few men tell him straight out about their difficulties in clear and accurate language. But many more are of the "try to figure out what I'm really talking about" school. They tell him that their wives haven't been happy since they started taking the medication. Some men use colorful euphemisms like "my noodle stays wet" and "my organ doesn't want to play," as well as others of a decidedly X-rated nature!

More frustrating are the men who tell Henry at their next cardiology clinic visit that they stopped taking their beta-blocker on their own shortly after they started it—but won't tell the reason why they stopped it. Now he has to work with a patient whose blood pressure, CAD, or other serious cardiac problem hasn't been treated adequately since the last office visit. This also leaves Henry in the dark about whether he should prescribe a lower dose of the medication that's been stopped or to try a different medication.

The lesson to be learned from this is to tell your doctor if you have sexual side effects from any medication. As we've stressed before, good physicians become desensitized to discussing anything that's biological —including sex. They won't be embarrassed and they shouldn't make you feel embarrassed if you discuss these problems with them.

Other Heart Medications and Sexual Dysfunction

Although beta-blockers are most (in)famous for causing sexual side effects, other medications commonly used to treat heart disease and hypertension can also do it. Diuretics ("water pills") are used to treat fluid retention from many causes, including congestive heart failure. Hydrochlorothiazide is used either by itself or in pills containing it along with another heart medication, particularly those used to treat hypertension. Although uncommon, hydrochlorothiazide can cause impotence. Spironolactone is used in patients with severely weakened hearts. This medication can occasionally decrease libido and cause ED—you don't want to have sex and couldn't do it even if you did. Bumetanide, a potent diuretic, causes premature ejaculation in about one out of a thousand men.

Several other types of heart medications we've discussed in previous chapters can also cause sexual problems. Angiotensin-converting enzyme (ACE) inhibitors and angiotensin receptor blockers are two similar classes of heart medications used to treat hypertension, heart failure, mitral regurgitation, aortic regurgitation, and some patients with CAD. Both groups of medications are only rarely associated with sexual side effects. Clonidine and methyldopa are two similar medications used to treat hypertension. Clonidine has been associated with decreased libido and ED in about 3% of men taking it. Methyldopa can cause similar problems.

Flecainide, a medication used to treat certain types of abnormal heart rhythms, causes decreased libido in about 1% of men. Gemfibrozil, a medication used for lowering cholesterol, can also rarely cause ED. Digoxin, used to treat heart failure and abnormal heart rhythms like atrial fibrillation, can occasionally cause sexual dysfunction.

Some commonly used heart medications have no definite association with ED. For example, various kinds of "blood thinners" are used extensively in patients with cardiac problems. Aspirin is extremely useful in patients with CAD, especially at the time of a heart attack. It can also reduce the risk of stroke in patients with blockages in the arteries of their neck, as well as some patients with atrial fibrillation or atrial flutter.

Clopidogrel and, less commonly, ticlopidine are blood thinners used along with aspirin in some patients with heart attacks, CAD, and blockages in the arteries of the neck. Both clopidogrel and aspirin are routinely used for a period of months or longer after a person has a stent placed in a coronary artery. Clopidogrel and ticlopidine can also be used as a substitute for aspirin in patients who can't take this medication because aspirin causes significant side effects like wheezing or stomach ulcers in them.

Warfarin (Coumadin) is used to reduce risk of stroke in patients with mechanical heart valves or atrial fibrillation. Warfarin is also used with many other heart problems and medical conditions to prevent blood clots from forming or to treat blood clots if they do occur.

Aspirin, clopidogrel, ticlopidine, and warfarin do not directly interfere with having sex. However, they could increase the chance of bleeding if one or both partners are too "rough" during sex. If that happens, we suggest being a little more gentle.

Nitrates are useful for treating angina in patients with CAD. They are also used to treat heart failure. This class of medications includes nitroglycerin in the form of a paste, patch, pill, and a tiny tablet or spray under the tongue. Isosorbide mononitrate and isosorbide dinitrate also belong to this class. Nitrates themselves only rarely cause sexual dysfunction. However, they can indirectly cause a serious problem in men who already have ED. If these men use nitrates, they cannot safely take several important medications used to treat ED.

Medications Used to Treat Sexual Dysfunction
Fortunately, while some medications "take away," a few can actually "give." It would be hard to find a medication whose trade name is better known by the general public than Viagra. This medication, whose generic name is sildenafil, was the first of a new class of medications, "phosphodiesterase type 5 inhibitors," used to treat ED. Since its approval by the Food and Drug Administration in 1998, Viagra has been a much more popular way of dealing with ED than the alternative medications or mechanical means we'll discuss later.

Recently Viagra has been joined by two similar medications, vardenafil (Levitra) and tadalafil (Cialis). The "success" rate of all these medications is similar. They differ primarily only in how long their effects last. Viagra and Levitra are effective for up to about 4 hours after being taken, while Cialis works for up to 36 hours. Another difference is that the way Cialis is absorbed into the body isn't affected by eating, while eating a fatty meal can delay absorption of Viagra and Levitra. It is suggested that Viagra be taken on an empty stomach.

Side effects common to all three medications include headache, nasal congestion, and flushing. Viagra can cause temporary visual problems, while these are significantly less common with Levitra or Cialis. Back and muscle pains are more common with Cialis than with the other two medications.

None of these medications directly causes the penis to become erect. Instead they do their "elevating" work only after sexual stimulation occurs. This stimulation causes release of a chemical called nitric oxide. This chemical in turn causes production of "cyclic guanosine monophosphate." This substance relaxes the muscles and blood vessels in the penis, causing more blood to enter it and producing an erection. Viagra, Levitra, and Cialis all work by blocking an enzyme, phosphodiesterase type 5, that breaks down cyclic guanosine monophosphate. With more of this enzyme available, blood flow into the penis increases and the chances of achieving an erection become higher.

These three medications normally cause only a mild decrease in blood pressure and slight increase in heart rate. However, if a man takes Viagra, Levitra, or Cialis with a nitrate medication such as isosorbide or nitroglycerin, his blood pressure may fall to a dangerously low level and make him pass out—or perhaps even die. This is because nitrates also increase the amount of nitric oxide in the body, thus amplifying the effects of Viagra and its cohorts—including how much they drop a person's blood pressure.

Current recommendations are that no form of nitrate should be taken within at least 24 hours after using Viagra or Levitra or within at least 48 hours after using Cialis. If a man needs to take long-acting nitrates like isosorbide or is likely to need to take nitroglycerin under the tongue to treat chest pain, he should not use Viagra, Levitra, or Cialis.

Prazosin, doxazosin, and terazosin are medications —"alpha-blockers"—used to treat high blood pressure. These medications are also used to treat enlargement of the prostate in older men. Like nitrates, alpha-blockers can cause a serious drop in blood pressure with Viagra, Levitra, and Cialis, although this risk is lower than it is with nitrates. It is recommended that a dose of Viagra more than 25 mg should not be taken within four hours of taking an alpha-blocker. Levitra should not be taken with any alpha-blocker or with several heart medications used to treat arrhythmias, including quinidine, procainamide, amiodarone, and sotalol. Cialis should also not be used with alpha-blockers. It is also recommended that Cialis should be used with caution in men taking any of a wide variety of blood pressure medications, such as beta-blockers or ACE inhibitors, due to the risk of excessive fall in blood pressure.

Viagra, Levitra, and Cialis may also indirectly increase risk of heart attack or death by themselves in men with severe heart disease. This can occur by motivating these men to try to exert themselves to a higher level of activity during sex than they normally do in their usual activities. By doing this they may increase the amount of work their heart is asked to do beyond a safe level. It is suggested that Viagra, Levitra, and Cialis should be used cautiously or not at all in men who have had a heart attack, stroke, or life-threatening arrhythmia within the last six months; those whose blood pressure runs lower or much higher than normal; and those with severe heart failure or severe CAD. Later in this chapter we'll discuss how men with heart disease are evaluated to see when it is safe to take Viagra and similar medications.

Other Treatments for Sexual Dysfunction

If a person can't safely take Viagra, Levitra, or Cialis, other medications and techniques to achieve a successful erection are available. However, they require more effort and discomfort that just swallowing a pill. Alprostadil is a medicine that, like Viagra and similar medications, increases the flow of blood into the penis. The exact way alprostadil does this, however, is different from Viagra, Levitra, and Cialis. Even more different is the way alprostadil is given. It needs to be either injected through a needle into the base of the penis (ouch!) or inserted in the form of a tiny pellet a couple inches into the penis itself through the urethra (ouch again!).

Given either way, alprostadil can take up to about twenty minutes to start "working." Its effects last for about an hour. In its injectable form alprostadil is sometimes mixed with other "helpful" chemicals, like phentolamine or papaverine. Not surprisingly, whichever way it's given, the major side effect of using alprostadil is pain in the penis.

Although uncommon, ED can be associated with abnormally low levels of testosterone, the male sex hormone. Your doctor can do a blood test to check for this. Testosterone can be replaced using injections, patches, etc.

One treatment for ED that requires no medication is the use of a vacuum device. This method involves drawing blood into the penis by inserting it into a tube with a small manual or battery-powered pump attached. Using the pump creates a mild vacuum and draws blood into the penis. Once enough blood has been drawn into the penis to achieve an erection, a small ring or band is placed around the base of the penis just tight enough to maintain the erection. The tube and vacuum pump are then removed. After intercourse is finished—or no more than thirty minutes, whichever comes first—the ring is removed.

People taking blood thinners like warfarin should use this kind of vacuum device either cautiously or not at all, since it may cause swelling or bruising of the penis. Needless to say, this method should *not* be tried using any type of household electric vacuum cleaner. The potential complications might get your name in one of the tabloid newspapers or under an "Odd News" heading on the Internet. However, the cost of this fame would be much too painful.

As a measure of last resort, surgery can be done to place a "penile implant." There are two basic varieties of this device. One inserts metal or plastic rods into the penis, keeping it somewhat rigid all the time. These rods allow the penis to be bent upward into a position for intercourse.

The other type of penile implant is an "inflatable" device that allows the man to achieve an erection on demand. It consists of two cylinders placed within the penis and connected by tubes to a small pump inside the scrotum. This type of device usually includes a small reservoir holding several ounces of fluid that is implanted under muscles near the groin. The man squeezes the pump, sending fluid into the cylinders within the penis to expand them and produce an erection. Thus, instead of the normal situation of blood flowing into the penis to make it erect, this fluid flowing into the implanted cylinders does roughly the same thing. The penis does not elongate as much as with a normal erection. The implant does, however, maintain the erection until the man releases it by squeezing another part of the pump to drain fluid back into the reservoir.

Heart Disease and Sexual Dysfunction

The methods we've described for dealing with ED apply to healthy men as well as those with heart problems or other significant health issues. ED is particularly common in men with CAD and diseases that increase the risk of having CAD. These include diabetes, high cholesterol, hypertension, and peripheral arterial disease.

In fact, having ED by itself indicates a man is at increased risk of having CAD and other problems like stroke. This is because, in a significant number of men, ED is at least partly due to atherosclerosis of the arteries that supply blood to the penis, reducing blood flow there. The same risk factors that produced atherosclerosis there can, of course, also affect the arteries of the heart and cause CAD. It's possible that, in men who have both ED due to vascular disease and CAD, "symptoms" involving the penis may occur before they have chest pain or other evidence of heart disease.

Right now, it's uncertain whether the mere presence of ED is enough by itself to trigger a specific evaluation of the heart, such as a stress test, if a man doesn't have chest pain or other heart symptoms. However, ED can alert the physician to check if the man has other risk factors for both CAD and ED, such as diabetes or high cholesterol.

Several tests can be done to check for blockages or other problems with blood flow to the penis that could cause ED. An ultrasound test can be used to check for blockages in the blood supply to the penis. This ultrasound study uses the same principles for taking pictures and checking blood flow as the echocardiogram and Doppler tests we discussed in Chapter 8. Medications that normally increase blood flow in the arteries and veins to the penis can be given as part of the ultrasound test to see if the blood vessels respond the way they should. Occasionally an arteriogram—injecting dye into the arteries that supply the penis, similar to how a coronary angiogram is done—is used to directly look for blockages. Tests with very fancy and very long names—cavernosometry and cavernosography—can be used to assess blood flow in the penis.

We should also mention that, besides problems with its blood supply, abnormalities of the nerves that supply the penis can also cause ED. As we described in an Chapter 2, parasympathetic nerves originating in the spinal cord are needed to produce an erection, while sympathetic nerves trigger ejaculation. Abnormalities in the nervous system from the brain on down can disrupt this process. These abnormalities include stroke, spinal cord injury, Parkinson's disease, multiple sclerosis, and a disease that affects blood vessels and nerves, diabetes. Damage to the prostate gland related to cancer or surgery can also cause ED.

Evaluating the Safety of Sexual Activity
Men with heart problems and ED need to be evaluated to see if it is safe for them to use medications like Viagra or to have sex at all. The same thing applies to anyone else with heart disease, whether the person is a man without ED or a woman. Determining if a person with heart disease can safely have sex is based on whether he or she can perform the level of exertion needed to do it with a reasonable margin of safety.

The amount of exertion needed to perform sex is actually modest. Previous studies have shown that, during intercourse, the heart rate usually doesn't get higher than about 130 beats per minute. Systolic blood pressure doesn't usually rise above about 170 to 180 mm Hg. These peak values are usually reached and sustained only relatively briefly, at the time of orgasm. It's interesting to note that some of these studies were done with married medical students and physicians in training. These highly motivated young couples, willing to put out their all to advance medical science, wore devices to continuously monitor their heart rates and blood pressures during their intimate time together. (It certainly beats being "on call" at the hospital!)

Before orgasm, the amount of exertion needed to perform sexual intercourse is about 2 to 3 METs. One MET, or metabolic equivalent, is the amount of oxygen the body uses when a healthy person is sitting quietly. Other activities that require an energy level of 2 to 3 METs include playing the piano, walking at a rate of about 2 miles per hour, slow ballroom dancing, or watering the plants at home. At the time of orgasm the amount of energy needed is about 3 to 4 METs, assuming the person is with a familiar partner and in familiar surroundings. Activities equivalent to this level of exertion include walking at a rate of 3 to 4 miles per hour, calisthenics (done without using weights), vacuuming at home, or raking the lawn.

In unfamiliar surroundings or a more stressful situation, like an illicit liaison in a strange motel, the peak MET level may rise to 5 or 6 METs. The energy needed for this level of exertion is still only equivalent to chopping wood, riding a bicycle at a moderate speed, or fast ballroom dancing. However, the peak heart rate and blood pressure during sex are mildly higher than they are during other types of activities with a similar MET level. The peak heart rate and blood pressure during sex also tend to be higher in men with CAD than the "normal" values we gave previously. They may also be higher in people with hypertension and those who are not physically fit.

Assessing the Risk of Sex with Heart Disease

One method your doctor can use to decide how risky sex is for your heart is based on the Princeton Guidelines. These guidelines were developed in 1999 by a panel of experts meeting at Princeton University—hence the name. The Princeton Guidelines help doctors decide whether someone with known or suspected heart disease has a "low," "intermediate," or "high" risk of having heart problems with sex.

Using these guidelines, your doctor first identifies any risk factors you have for heart disease. These risk factors include your age (the older you are the higher the risk); being male or a postmenopausal female; hypertension; diabetes; obesity; smoking cigarettes; high cholesterol; and an inactive, "couch potato" lifestyle. You qualify for the low-risk category if you have only two or fewer of these risk factors for cardiovascular disease, excluding the one about being a male or postmenopausal female.

However, to make sure you really are in this low-risk category, your doctor also checks if you have any symptoms due to heart disease, such as chest pain (angina) or shortness of breath. Your doctor will ask if you have a history of a previous heart attack, stroke, heart valve problem, or peripheral arterial disease. Based on your history and physical examination, your doctor may order additional tests to check for these problems. These may include an echocardiogram, a stress test, or a coronary angiogram. If you have controlled hypertension; mild stable angina; a previous successful coronary angioplasty or coronary artery bypass graft surgery (CABG); a heart attack more than six to eight weeks ago; mild heart valve disease; or a history of decreased heart function or heart failure that doesn't cause any symptoms with normal activity, you also qualify for the low-risk category for sex. People who are at low risk based on these criteria can go ahead and have sex, from the heart standpoint, with a good margin of safety. Men in this category can, if needed, use medications like Viagra to treat ED. However, the precautions we discussed before about using nitrates, alpha-blockers, and certain other medications with Viagra, Levitra, and Cialis still apply. For example, if a man has been taking oral nitrates for angina, the doctor will need to taper it off and stop it if this can be done safely, perhaps replacing the oral nitrate with a different medication such as a calcium antagonist.

Also, to give an extra level of reassurance that it's safe to have sex, doing an exercise stress test after coronary artery angioplasty, CABG, or a heart attack may be prudent. If the exercise test shows a person can perform moderate exercise—at least 4 to 5 METs and preferably 5 to 6 METs or more—without developing myocardial ischemia (decreased blood flow to the heart muscle) or other problems, then it is most likely safe to resume sexual activity.

On the other hand, people found to be in the Princeton "intermediate" and "high" risk groups should *not* engage in sex or take ED medications until they've had additional evaluation and treatment. Intermediate risk means a person has three or more of the risk factors—once again, excluding gender—we described previously; moderate, stable angina; had a heart attack between two to six weeks ago; has decreased heart function or heart failure that causes shortness of breath or other symptoms only with normal or greater than normal activity; has peripheral arterial disease; or had a previous stroke.

People with intermediate risk need better control of their cardiovascular problems by adjusting their medications; improvement of their risk factors—for example, achieving good control of blood pressure; and further evaluation with a stress test, coronary angiogram, or other tests. If, after being evaluated and treated, these people now qualify for the low-risk category, then they too can get the "go ahead" for sex.

People in the high-risk category have angina that's unstable or not controlled despite good medical or other treatment; uncontrolled high blood pressure; symptoms from heart failure even when they do light activity or are just sitting still; a heart attack or stroke less than two weeks ago; serious arrhythmias; certain types of cardiomyopathy; or moderate to severe heart valve disease. These people definitely need to be fully evaluated and stabilized before they can safely have sex. If, with treatment, they improve to the point of meeting the criteria for the low-risk category, they too can resume sex.

A person can do several simple things to reduce the amount of work the heart has to do during sex. One of them is to wait at least one to three hours after finishing a meal before having sex. The heart has to work harder to supply blood to the stomach, intestines, pancreas and other organs in your abdomen while you're digesting your food. It's best to wait until these organs have done most of their job before having sex. Also, having sex when you're relaxed, free from any increased stress from your normal activities or from dealing with problems, will also give the heart more reserve.

Ultimately, it's important to talk with your doctor about what medications are best for maintaining a healthy sex life—specifically, which medications can be safely used and which should be avoided. Whether you've just been found to have CAD or another heart problem, or you are recuperating from a heart attack or heart surgery, your doctor will use the kinds of principles we've discussed to advise you when you can safely resume sex.

Chapter 12 Summary
- ♥ "Erectile dysfunction" or ED means that a man is unable on a particular occasion to have an erection sufficient to perform sexual intercourse.

- ♥ Erectile dysfunction can be caused by beta-blockers and other heart medications.

- ♥ Medications, devices, and procedures are available to treat erectile dysfunction. Discuss options to treat erectile dysfunction with your doctor or other healthcare provider.

- ♥ Many men who are either healthy or have heart disease can safely take Viagra, Levitra, and Cialis to treat erectile dysfunction. Nitrates should never be taken with Viagra, Levitra, or Cialis.

- ♥ Men and women with known or suspected heart disease should be evaluated to determine how safe it is for them to have sex.

Chapter 13: Oh, Baby!
Pregnancy and Heart Disease

Chapter Preview:
Pregnancy and the Normal Heart
  Effects of pregnancy on heart rate and blood pressure
Pregnancy and Palpitations
  Premature atrial and ventricular contractions
  Effects of labor and delivery on the heart
Peripartum Cardiomyopathy
  Heart failure during pregnancy
Pregnancy and High Blood Pressure
  High blood pressure during pregnancy
  Preeclampsia and eclampsia
Pregnancy and Coronary Artery Disease
  Management of coronary artery disease during pregnancy
  Risk of heart attack during pregnancy
Pregnancy and Congenital Heart Disease
  Special risks in women with congenital heart disease
  Patent ductus arteriosus and coarctation of the aorta
Pregnancy and Severe Congenital Heart Disease
  Tetralogy of Fallot
  Transposition of the great vessels
Pregnancy and Pulmonary Hypertension
  Pulmonary hypertension caused by congenital heart disease
  Ebstein's anomaly
  Corrected transposition of the great vessels
  Eisenmenger's syndrome
  Primary pulmonary hypertension
Pregnancy and Myocarditis
  Myocarditis and heart failure

Pregnancy and Arrhythmias
    Premature atrial or ventricular contractions as signs of other medical problems
    Pregnancy and paroxysmal supraventricular tachycardia
Pregnancy and Heart Valve Disease
    Medical treatment of heart valve disease
    Procedures and surgery for heart valve disease
Pregnancy and Artificial Heart Valves
    Tissue versus mechanical heart valves with pregnancy
Pregnancy and Heart Medications
    Categories of medications based on risk to the baby during pregnancy
Pregnancy and Warfarin
    Indications for warfarin during pregnancy
    Risks of warfarin to the unborn baby
    Heparin and other alternatives to warfarin during pregnancy
    Breastfeeding and heart medications
Pregnancy and Cardiac Testing
    Tests with low risk to mother and baby during pregnancy
    Radiation risks of coronary angiography and other heart tests

WHEN A FERTILE man and a fertile women have unprotected sex, there's a certain chance their liaison will produce a baby. Even if you weren't familiar with all the details of this process before reading Chapter 2, the basic concept behind the "birds and the bees" is hardly a secret. Pregnancy is a major, hopefully joyful milestone in a woman's life. But if the mother-to-be has heart disease, pregnancy can be a serious matter.

Pregnancy and the Normal Heart

Morning sickness, back pain, swelling in the ankles, shortness of breath, fatigue—these are some of the physical stresses the expectant mother has to cope with during even the most normal pregnancy. The heart also has to work harder. Heart rate starts to increase early during pregnancy as the woman's body adapts to provide energy and nutrition to the new life growing within her. From the first three months of pregnancy until delivery, a woman's resting heart rate can be well above the usual upper range of 100 beats per minute. Henry has had pregnant women referred to him for cardiac consultation because they've had heart rates as high as 100 beats per minute when they are resting and over 170 beats per minute when they are active. These heart rates can be and usually are normal during pregnancy.

While the expectant mother's heart rate usually increases during pregnancy, both her systolic and diastolic blood pressures are generally below normal during the first six months after conception. Both types of blood pressure then rise to or above normal near the time of delivery. If blood pressure drops too low, it can cause lightheadedness, nausea, weakness, or even passing out—"syncope." Early in pregnancy, these symptoms are most likely to occur when a woman who's been lying down or sitting stands up suddenly. This is because blood pressure normally falls temporarily when a person first stands up. If the woman's blood pressure is already fairly low when she's lying down or sitting, when she stands up her blood pressure may drop too low to supply enough blood to her brain and the rest of her body. If she does feel lightheaded or have other symptoms, she should sit or lie back down again.

Later in the pregnancy, when a woman lies on her back, the weight of her enlarged uterus can compress the inferior vena cava, the large vein that carries blood from the lower part of the body back to the heart. This makes blood pressure drop because the heart is getting less blood, again causing potential problems with lightheadedness and passing out. Generations of women have discovered the treatment for this problem on their own—lay on your side, to shift the uterus away from the inferior vena cava so it's not being compressed.

Pregnancy and Palpitations
From very early in pregnancy to the time of delivery, the total amount of blood the heart pumps each minute, called the "cardiac output," increases significantly. Because the heart really is working harder than usual, women may feel palpitations due to their more forceful heartbeats. It's also normal for them to experience "extra" heartbeats—premature atrial contractions (PACs) and premature ventricular contractions (PVCs). As we discussed in Chapter 6, PACs and PVCs are beats that occur earlier than a person's normal heartbeats—hence the "premature" part of their name. They are caused by electrical impulses originating in an abnormal location, either in an atrium (PACs) or a ventricle (PVCs). A woman may notice them because they occur earlier than normal or because the normal beat after them is more forceful than usual.

While PACs and PVCs can be a sign of underlying heart disease or other health problems such as abnormal thyroid function, even when they occur frequently they are usually *not* associated with any other problems. These abnormal heartbeats usually disappear within months after delivery.

Not surprisingly, the biggest strain on the heart occurs at the time of labor. Pain, anxiety, and the contractions of the uterus itself make heart rate, blood pressure, and cardiac output increase dramatically during vaginal delivery. A cesarean section ("C-section") generally puts less but still significant stress on the heart. Right after delivery, the shrinking uterus no longer compresses the inferior vena cava, and blood from the uterus itself shifts back into the mother's bloodstream. All this "extra" blood returning to the heart can, for several hours after the baby's birth, make the mother's heart work even harder than it did during labor. Later, the heart rate, blood pressure, and cardiac output decrease toward normal. However, they may not return to pre-pregnancy levels for as long as six months after delivery.

The vast majority of healthy women are obviously able to tolerate all the extra work the heart has to do during pregnancy. However, when the heart or major blood vessels are abnormal, pregnancy can be a very serious business. You may be wondering just how common this problem actually is. After all, pregnancy is something that happens to younger women, and most heart disease occurs at ages beyond the child-bearing years.

Unfortunately, some forms of heart disease are actually *more* commonly seen in younger people, particularly those involving congenital problems (birth defects) and abnormal heart valves caused by rheumatic fever. Even some types of heart disease that are more frequently present in older women occur in a significant number of younger ones. The average age of menopause in American women is now about 51 years old. This means that some premenopausal women, particularly those in their thirties and forties, will have significant risk factors for heart disease. These risk factors include diabetes, high blood pressure, smoking, use of oral contraceptives, cancers requiring radiation treatments to the chest, and so on. Some of these women will develop coronary artery disease (CAD), heart failure, and other serious problems that can substantially increase the risk of pregnancy.

Peripartum Cardiomyopathy
Even previously healthy women can develop heart disease for the first time during pregnancy. Peripartum cardiomyopathy is a form of heart disease that causes enlargement of the heart and weakening of the heart muscle. It occurs at a rate of about 1 out of 3000 to 1 out of 4000 in women who give birth to a live baby. Peripartum cardiomyopathy can begin anywhere from the middle of pregnancy to as long as five months after delivery, but it is seen most commonly shortly after the baby is delivered. Peripartum cardiomyopathy is most likely to occur during a first or second pregnancy and in women more than 30 years old. Symptoms that women normally experience during pregnancy—shortness of breath, ankle swelling, palpitations, etc.—are more severe with peripartum cardiomyopathy.

Peripartum cardiomyopathy can cause heart failure. It often requires treatment with medications. Heart function returns to normal in more than half of women within six months after delivery. However, in a significant minority of women, heart function doesn't improve. Heart function may even deteriorate to the point where a heart transplant is needed to avoid death from severe heart failure or life-threatening arrhythmias. Women who recover completely from peripartum cardiomyopathy have a small but significant risk of it recurring during a later pregnancy. The risk of death in these women, however, is very low. On the other hand, those whose hearts were permanently damaged due to peripartum cardiomyopathy are likely to suffer further heart damage with another pregnancy. These women also have about a one out of four chance of dying during a later pregnancy.

Pregnancy and High Blood Pressure
High blood pressure (hypertension) is a common problem that a woman may have even before she becomes pregnant. Blood pressure during pregnancy should preferably be lower than 140/90 millimeters of mercury (mm Hg). It is especially important to control blood pressure during pregnancy if the expectant mother has diabetes, abnormal kidney function, or other serious medical problems. Uncontrolled hypertension can cause kidney failure, stroke, and both low birth weight and premature delivery of the baby. As we'll discuss later, several blood pressure medications are preferably not used during pregnancy due to their potential risks to the baby. However, most blood pressure medications can be used with reasonable safety for both mother and baby.

Pregnancy itself can cause hypertension. It can begin as early as five months into the pregnancy and typically resolves by six weeks after delivery. A blood pressure of more than 140/90 mm Hg on two separate readings at least six hours apart indicates hypertension is present. The risk to both the mother and baby is significantly increased if hypertension is associated with increased protein in the urine, a condition called "preeclampsia."

Preeclampsia occurs in about 5% of pregnancies in American women. The reason why preeclampsia occurs is not completely understood. The risk of developing preeclampsia is greatest in women less than 20 years old. A woman with preeclampsia may also have abdominal pain, blurred vision, and abnormal blood tests. Preeclampsia may progress further to eclampsia, with occurrence of seizures and coma, as well as potentially permanent injury or death to mother and baby. Eclampsia occurs in about 0.2% of pregnancies.

Mild cases of preeclampsia are usually managed with bed rest and medications to lower the blood pressure. The baby is delivered at or a few weeks before the due date. Severe preelampsia may require delivery of the baby up to several months before the due date, if testing shows the baby weighs enough to be delivered safely. While medications are of some help in treating severe preeclampsia and eclampsia, the most definitive treatment to prevent injury or death to the mother and baby is to deliver the baby. Both preeclampsia and eclampsia usually resolve within a day after delivery.

Pregnancy and Coronary Artery Disease

Cardiologists occasionally have pregnant women with known CAD referred to them. Some of these women have had angioplasty or bypass surgery before. Except for avoiding certain medications that can harm the baby (more on these medicines later), their treatment generally remains the same as it was before they came pregnant. They continue to need good control of blood pressure and to avoid smoking. Managing high cholesterol can be difficult, since LDL cholesterol and triglycerides normally rise significantly during pregnancy. Some standard cholesterol-lowering medicines can also harm the baby.

Most pregnant women with CAD will do well with vaginal delivery, supported by good pain relief and use of oxygen. If they develop chest pain or other signs the heart may not be getting enough blood, a cesarean section can be done to reduce their overall stress and shorten the time it takes to deliver the baby.

Fortunately, the risk of having a heart attack during pregnancy and delivery is low. Women who have a heart attack usually have it during the last third of pregnancy. While a heart attack can occur even in teenagers, the risk is greater when the mother is in her mid-thirties or older or if she has had multiple pregnancies. Though it's usually due to CAD alone, a heart attack can also be caused by other problems. These include a coronary artery going into spasm, a new blood clot forming in a coronary artery, or a spontaneous tear (dissection) in the inner wall of a coronary artery that cuts off blood flow.

Evaluating chest pain during pregnancy in a woman with or without known CAD can be challenging. While many standard heart tests, such as EKGs and echocardiograms, are harmless to both mother and baby, others are not. Exercise stress tests can cause abnormal slowing of the baby's heart rate. The mother may also have difficulty performing a high enough level of exercise to evaluate the heart.

Myocardial perfusion imaging and coronary angiography expose the baby to low but potentially harmful levels of radiation. Radiation exposure during pregnancy can increase a baby's risk of having birth defects and developing cancer later during childhood. Myocardial perfusion imaging and coronary angiography are therefore reserved for situations in which the suspicion of CAD and the need for possible angioplasty or bypass surgery are high enough to justify the risk to both mother and baby.

Pregnancy and Congenital Heart Disease

A pregnant mother with significant congenital heart disease—abnormalities in the heart chambers, valves, or major blood vessels present from birth—has an increased risk of developing heart failure, hypertension, and arrhythmias. She is more likely to have miscarriages and has an increased risk of dying during delivery. Her baby is more likely to have a lower birth weight, be born prematurely, and to have congenital heart disease itself.

The degree of risk to the mother and her baby depends on the type of congenital heart disease she has and how severe it is. The most common abnormalities are only rarely associated with serious complications to either mother or baby during pregnancy. They include a small atrial septal defect—an abnormal opening in the tissue separating the right atrium and the left atrium—and a bicuspid aortic valve—the valve has two leaflets instead of the normal three—without significant narrowing of the valve.

Some types of congenital heart defects may be only mildly abnormal in one woman but severely abnormal in another. For example, a mild congenital narrowing (stenosis) of the pulmonic valve is usually not associated with any problems during pregnancy. However, the pulmonic valve can also be severely narrowed, significantly reducing blood flow to the lungs and to the rest of the body. This increases the risk of death for both mother and baby. A mother with severe pulmonic stenosis may have chest pain, increased shortness of breath, or may pass out. She may require a procedure during pregnancy to open the valve using a catheter with an inflatable balloon on the end—balloon valvotomy.

Women with a patent ductus arteriosus (PDA) have a blood vessel that causes abnormal blood flow from the aorta to the pulmonary artery. They usually tolerate pregnancy well if the amount of blood flow between these two major arteries is small. However, if the amount of blood flow through the PDA is too great it can overload the right side of the heart. In the most severe cases, the direction of blood flow can reverse, causing oxygen-poor venous blood to go from the pulmonary artery into the aorta. This reduces the amount of oxygen the rest of the body gets. If needed, the PDA can be closed off. A cardiologist with specialized training can use special catheters to insert a "plug" into the PDA and block it off. A cardiovascular surgeon can also do an operation to tie the PDA off.

Coarctation of the aorta is a congenital defect in which a small part of the aorta is "pinched" or narrowed to some degree. This area of narrowing occurs high in the chest, a short distance after the aorta makes a U-turn from where it attaches to the left ventricle and heads down toward the lower part of the body. Coarctation of the aorta is associated with increased risk of heart failure, hypertension, and rupture of the aorta. It is also very commonly associated with a bicuspid aortic valve, which in turn has an increased risk of infection and becoming narrowed.

Coarctation of the aorta may be severe enough to be life-threatening in infants and children. However, milder cases may produce no definite symptoms and not be detected until adulthood. When coarctation of the aorta is found, surgery is indicated to repair it. However, if it is first discovered when a woman is pregnant, medical treatment to keep blood pressure under good control is usually the best choice until delivery. Coarctation of the aorta is also associated with aneurysms (widening) of certain arteries in the brain. These aneurysms can rupture during pregnancy and cause a stroke.

Pregnancy and Severe Congenital Heart Disease
Some types of congenital heart disease are very severe. Until surgical procedures to improve survival were developed several decades ago, the chances of a girl with one of them surviving to puberty were remote. Now, with surgery these same girls can survive to adulthood. However, the heart is still abnormal enough to increase risk during pregnancy.

Several serious congenital heart defects involve major abnormalities in the relationships between the chambers of the heart and the two main blood vessels arising from it, the pulmonary artery and the aorta. In tetralogy of Fallot, there is an abnormal opening in the tissue that separates the right and left ventricle—a "ventricular septal defect." The right ventricle is also abnormally thick (hypertrophied). The aorta comes off the heart between the right and left ventricles, rather than just from the left ventricle. There is also a partial obstruction between the right ventricle and the pulmonary artery.

In uncorrected transposition of the great vessels, the aorta comes off the right ventricle and the pulmonary artery arises from the left ventricle. For a baby with this particular problem to live, there must also be some type of abnormal blood flow between the two sides of the heart, such as an opening between its two upper or lower chambers.

Pregnancy and Pulmonary Hypertension
Severe congenital heart defects such as tetralogy of Fallot and uncorrected transposition of the great

vessels cause two problems that markedly increase the risk to both mother and baby during pregnancy. First, a significant amount of oxygen-poor blood from the right side of the heart bypasses the lungs and mixes with blood going out to the rest of the body. This produces a "cyanotic" appearance, with the tips of fingers and toes appearing blue due to lack of oxygen in the blood. Second, the right side of the heart commonly fails and pressures in the arteries of the lung rise above normal—"pulmonary hypertension."

Women with congenital heart disease severe enough to cause these two problems have trouble supplying enough oxygen to their body to supply their own needs, much less their baby's needs. Up to 40% of these women die within a few weeks after delivery. This risk is so high that they are advised not to become pregnant. However, if surgery to at least partially correct severe congenital heart disease like tetralogy of Fallot is done during childhood, pulmonary hypertension and other problems associated with these heart abnormalities may not develop or be only mild. In that case, the risk to the woman and her baby during pregnancy may be relatively low.

Several other types of congenital heart disease seen in women of childbearing age can, if severe enough, also eventually cause pulmonary hypertension. In Ebstein's anomaly, the tricuspid valve is abnormal. This valve is displaced downward into the right ventricle and can have significant leakage—tricuspid regurgitation. Over time the right ventricle may fail and pulmonary hypertension can develop. The average age Ebstein's anomaly is diagnosed is during the middle of the teenage years.

In corrected transposition of the great vessels, the right ventricle and left ventricle have switched places.

What is anatomically the right ventricle is where the left ventricle should be, pumping blood into the aorta. The anatomic left ventricle is where the right ventricle should be, pumping blood into the pulmonary artery. The right ventricle isn't designed to pump against the much higher blood pressures normally present in the aorta compared to the pulmonary artery. Eventually, the right ventricle can fail, causing both heart failure and pulmonary hypertension. Pregnancy can be tolerated reasonably well, however, if pulmonary hypertension hasn't developed.

Both an atrial septal defect and a ventricular septal defect initially involve blood passing from the left side of the heart to its right side. Blood flows in that direction because the pressures on the left side of the heart are normally higher than on the right side. If the size of an atrial septal defect or ventricular septal defect is small, the right ventricle can pump out the "extra" amount of blood it's getting from the left side of heart without any significant problem. Women with a small atrial septal defect or a very small ventricular septal defect typically do not have increased risk during pregnancy.

However, if the atrial septal defect or ventricular septal defect is large enough, the amount of blood getting to the right ventricle may be more than it can handle. If surgery to repair the defect isn't done before this happens, over a period of years the right ventricle can eventually fail. Pressures rise in the right ventricle and the pulmonary arteries due to all this extra blood flowing through them. The person develops gradually worsening pulmonary hypertension.

If pulmonary hypertension becomes severe enough, the pressure on the right side of the heart can actually exceed that on the left side—a very abnormal state of affairs. This causes "Eisenmenger's syndrome." The person becoming cyanotic, due to oxygen-poor blood from the right side of the heart mixing with blood on the left side. Common symptoms includes shortness of breath, limited ability to exercise, coughing up blood, and stroke due to blood clots passing from the right side of the heart to the left side. In a pregnant woman, Eisenmenger's syndrome is associated with a very high risk of death for both mother and baby.

Pulmonary hypertension can also be caused by many conditions other than severe congenital heart disease. It can be a complication of any type of severe lung disease. These diseases of the lung include ones that can be seen in young women, like cystic fibrosis, sarcoidosis, system lupus erythematosus (SLE, or "lupus"), use of certain weight-loss medications, or any condition that caused large areas of the lung to be damaged due to blood clots in its arteries. Heart failure involving the left side of the heart, as well as severe mitral or aortic valve disease, especially severe mitral stenosis, can also cause pulmonary hypertension.

In a small percentage of people with pulmonary hypertension, no cause can be found for it. This condition, "primary pulmonary hypertension," is most common in young women, with an average age at diagnosis of 36 years. It produces shortness of breath, fatigue, and chest pain. These symptoms can worsen during pregnancy. The risk of death to a mother with primary pulmonary hypertension is as high as when pulmonary hypertension is caused by severe congenital heart disease.

Overall, pulmonary hypertension from any cause increases the risk of death to both mother and baby. Mild pulmonary hypertension is associated with only mild risk, but the risks are very high with severe pulmonary hypertension—particularly that due to congenital heart disease.

Pregnancy and Myocarditis

Infections that damage heart muscle and valves can also seriously increase risk during pregnancy. Myocarditis, an infection of the heart muscle usually caused by a virus, can occur at any age. While most cases cause only mild or no symptoms and don't significantly damage the heart, occasionally it can cause permanent, severe injury to the heart and produce heart failure. Most women respond well to treatment with appropriate medications and close monitoring during pregnancy and delivery.

Rarely, heart failure is so severe after myocarditis develops that heart transplantation is needed. Although the number of women who've become pregnant after heart transplantation due to any kind of heart disease is small, their overall risk of death during pregnancy and delivery has not been higher than normal. However, women with heart transplants are somewhat more likely to have problems with hypertension and infections. Their babies also tend to have smaller birth weights and premature deliveries.

Pregnancy and Arrhythmias

In women without known heart disease, serious arrhythmias during pregnancy or delivery are unusual. The single PACs and PVCs we talked about before are common. However, they are rarely associated with any problems to the mother or baby except to give her palpitations. A Holter monitor or event monitor can be used to see how frequently PACs and PVCs occur and if any other types of arrhythmias are present. Laboratory tests to check for low or high thyroid function and other abnormalities that could worsen the palpitations can be checked. If there is a suspicion palpitations might be due to peripartum cardiomyopathy or some other significant heart problem, others tests such as an echocardiogram can also be ordered.

Even in otherwise healthy women, the risk of having one type of abnormal fast rhythm, paroxysmal supraventricular tachycardia (PSVT), may mildly increase during pregnancy. This arrhythmia makes the heart rate suddenly jump to 150 to 250 beats per minute—fast enough to significantly reduce blood flow to both the mother and baby. PSVT may go away by itself, or the mother may be able to stop it by straining as if she were having a bowel movement. If PSVT persists, a trip to the emergency room for an intravenous medication such as adenosine or even an electrical shock to the chest might be needed to treat it. Fortunately, the medications typically used to treat PSVT are short-acting and carry little risk to either mother or baby. Even electrical shocks to the chest are reasonably safe during pregnancy, although they are used only if necessary.

Pregnancy and Heart Valve Disease
Heart valve problems can also increase a woman's risk during pregnancy. Mitral stenosis, due predominantly to previous rheumatic fever, is seen in women of childbearing age. As we discussed in chapter 6, mitral stenosis can cause shortness of breath, coughing up blood, atrial fibrillation, and heart failure. These symptoms are likely to worsen during the course of pregnancy in a woman with moderate to severe mitral stenosis, at least partly due to the normal increase in heart rate that occurs with pregnancy. Fortunately, the risk of death in a mother with mitral stenosis is low.

Mitral stenosis can be treated during pregnancy with diuretics and beta-blockers. Digoxin can also be used to reduce heart rate if atrial fibrillation is present.

Balloon valvotomy can be used to treat severe mitral stenosis if the mother's symptoms aren't adequately controlled with medicines alone. Mitral valve replacement during pregnancy is reserved for only the most extreme cases. Mitral stenosis is also associated with premature birth and low birth weight in the baby. Most mothers with mitral stenosis can have a normal vaginal delivery and use an epidural anesthetic.

Aortic stenosis, either congenital or due to rheumatic fever, is uncommon in young women. A mild to moderate degree of aortic stenosis is usually tolerated well in pregnant women. However, women with severe aortic stenosis have a significant chance of having new or worsened symptoms of shortness of breath, passing out (syncope), heart failure, and chest pain. These symptoms are brought on or made worse by the normal changes in blood pressure and heart function that occur during pregnancy, which make the effects of aortic stenosis worse.

Medical therapy for aortic stenosis is limited, since the basic problem is a mechanical one—narrowing of the valve—that requires a mechanical solution—open it up or replace it. Medications, like diuretics used to treat heart failure, can only deal with this problem indirectly. If a pregnant woman has severe symptoms that don't respond well enough to medications, balloon valvotomy can be tried as a means to at least temporarily help her. In the most severe cases, aortic valve replacement can be done during the pregnancy as a measure of last resort.

Women with moderate and even severe mitral regurgitation or aortic regurgitation usually tolerate pregnancy well. Unlike women with aortic or mitral stenosis, the normal changes in heart function and blood pressure seen in pregnancy tend to reduce the amount of valve regurgitation. Women with symptoms like shortness of breath with their mitral or aortic regurgitation can usually be treated with medications. These include diuretics and medications like hydralazine that further lower blood pressure to an optimal range. Valve surgery during pregnancy is only rarely needed for women with mitral or aortic regurgitation.

Pregnancy and Artificial Heart Valves
If a young woman should require heart valve replacement before or during pregnancy, the same issues regarding what type of valve is used— mechanical valve versus tissue valve—described in an earlier chapter also apply. A person with a tissue (bioprosthetic) valve doesn't normally need to take "blood thinners" such as warfarin. On the other hand, tissue valves are much less durable than mechanical valves, especially in young people. They are also more likely to deteriorate and eventually need to be replaced again. Pregnancy itself may, in fact, accelerate deterioration of a tissue valve.

However, mechanical heart valves can cause several serious problems during pregnancy. Women with a mechanical valve need to take some kind of blood thinner to prevent blood clots from forming on the artificial valve. However, blood thinners increase the woman's chance of having excessive bleeding, particularly at the time of delivery. Pregnancy itself may increase the chance of blood clots forming on the valve and the valve malfunctioning even when the mother is taking an appropriate dose of the blood thinner. As we'll talk about soon, the standard blood thinner used, warfarin, also presents unique risks to her baby.

Pregnancy and Heart Medications

Mother and baby share a single blood supply. If the mother takes a medication, the baby will, to some degree, also get some of it. The basic rule for giving medicines to a pregnant woman is to give as few medicines as possible and to give them at the lowest dose needed to help the mother without harming the baby.

Early in pregnancy the baby's brain, internal organs, and limbs are just starting to develop and are most vulnerable to injury. Some medications can cause birth defects if the mother takes them then.

Later in pregnancy the baby's major body parts have fully developed and are just growing larger. Some medicines taken at that time can cause harm by causing too strong an effect on the baby, due to his or her much smaller size compared to the mother. For example, a dose of propranolol that causes only mild slowing of heart rate and lowering of blood pressure in the mother can produce significantly higher levels of that medicine in the baby. This could cause the baby's heart rate and blood pressure to fall dangerously low.

The Food and Drug Administration (FDA) has five categories for how risky it is to the baby for a pregnant woman to take a particular medication. Some medications fall into more than one category, with increased risk early in pregnancy but not later, or vice versa.

Category A medications have the lowest level of risk. Scientific studies haven't shown that these medicines harm the baby when the mother takes them during pregnancy. These medications include levothyroxine, used to treat low thyroid function;

ferrous sulfate (iron) tablets for treating anemia; and vitamin pills with standard doses of vitamin B and vitamin C. Unfortunately, none of our standard heart medications fall into this category with the lowest risk.

A medicine is in Category B if scientific studies using pregnant female animals, such as mice, have not shown that the medicine harms their developing babies, but there are no reports whether or not the medicine hurts a human baby if the mother takes it during pregnancy. A medicine is also listed in Category B if research shows it can hurt a pregnant female animal's babies, but studies have not shown that the medicine hurts a human baby if the mother uses it during pregnancy. Amiloride, a type of diuretic ("water pill"), and methyldopa, a medicine used to treat high blood pressure, are in Category B. A more commonly used diuretic, hydrochlorothiazide, is in this category when it's used during the last six months of pregnancy. However, when it is taken during the first three months of pregnancy, hydrochlorothiazide may cause birth defects and is in a higher-risk category (see below).

A medicine is classified as Category C if scientific studies have shown that it can sometimes harm unborn animal babies when it is given to pregnant female animals, but there aren't any studies to see if the medicine harms a human baby if the mother takes it during pregnancy. A medicine is also in Category C if there are no adequate studies testing its possible harm to either animal or human babies. Many heart medications are in Category C. They include digoxin; nitrates, such as isosorbide and nitroglycerin; and some calcium antagonists like diltiazem, verapamil, nifedipine, and nicardipine. Certain beta-blockers, such as propranolol, carvedilol, metoprolol, nadolol, and bisoprolol, are also in Category C. So are several medications used to treat arrhythmias, including flecainide, propafenone, procainamide, and quinidine.

Aspirin is a Category C medication when the mother takes it during the first six months of pregnancy. However, during the last three months of pregnancy, aspirin is the next higher risk category, Category D, if it's taken at a usual dose of 325 mg or more daily. This is because aspirin is more likely to hurt an unborn baby during the last three months of pregnancy than when the mother takes it during the first six months after conception.

Category D medicines are known to sometimes cause harm to a human baby if the mother takes it during pregnancy. However, these medicines may be used in certain circumstances when the overall benefit to the mother—and, perhaps, indirectly the baby—outweighs that risk. Amiodarone is used to treat abnormal heart rhythms. This medication can reduce thyroid function in the baby. Amiodarone has also been associated with premature birth and birth defects. Atenolol, a beta-blocker, is also in Category D. So is aspirin, if a pregnant woman takes it at a dose of 325 mg or more daily during the last three months of pregnancy.

ACE inhibitors such as captopril, lisinopril, or benazepril and angiotensin receptor blockers like irbesartan, olmesartan, or candesartan are in Category D if they are taken during the last six months of pregnancy. Both types of medications are currently listed as having lower risk—Category C—during the first three months of pregnancy. However, a recent report in the June 8, 2006 issue of the *New England Journal of Medicine* showed that ACE inhibitors taken during the first three months of pregnancy significantly increases the baby's risk of having serious birth defects involving the heart and nervous system. It is possible that taking ACE inhibitors early during pregnancy may be reclassified to a higher risk category if further studies confirm this risk.

Category X medications are known to cause harm to the baby. Their risk to the baby outweighs any possible benefit. In other words, if at all possible a pregnant woman should *not* take a Category X medicine. Unfortunately, most cholesterol-lowering medications—statins (such as atorvastatin and simvastatin), niacin, and eztimibe—fall into this category. For example, statins have been reported to cause problems with bone development in the baby. Amlodipine and felodipine, two commonly used calcium antagonists, are also in Category X.

Pregnancy and Warfarin
Warfarin is a category X medicine that presents a particularly difficult management problem during pregnancy. This particular "blood thinner"—more technically called an "anticoagulant"—is strongly indicated in certain heart conditions to reduce the chance of blood clots forming. These blood clots can potentially cause stroke or other problems. Warfarin is especially needed when the mother has a mechanical heart valve to prevent the valve from forming clots that could keep the heart valve from working right or cause a stroke.

However, taking warfarin during the first three months of pregnancy carries a significant risk of birth defects and miscarriage. When used between the first six to twelve weeks of pregnancy, this medicine can produce "warfarin embryopathy." The baby can be born with specific abnormalities such as a small malformed nose, cleft lip, calcium deposits in the growth plates of the arms and legs, or obstruction of the airway. Less commonly, warfarin can also cause a variety of serious defects in the baby's heart and other internal organs.

The risk to the baby is lower when warfarin is used during the last six months of pregnancy. However, it can still cause bleeding within the baby's head, reduced growth of brain tissue, blindness, mental retardation, and other serious problems.

Another anticoagulant, heparin, can be used instead of warfarin to significantly reduce the direct risk to the baby. In its usual "unfractionated" form, heparin is a Category C medication. "Fractionated" forms of heparin such as enoxaparin and dalteparin are in Category B. However, unlike warfarin, heparin cannot be given as a pill. Unfractionated heparin must be given either as a continuous intravenous infusion or by injections under the skin—the same way insulin shots are given. It can be difficult to regulate the dose of unfractionated heparin over the many months of pregnancy to make sure the mother's blood is neither too "thin," increasing the risk of bleeding, nor too "thick," increasing the risk of blood clots. It is easier to regulate the dose of warfarin.

Fractionated types of heparin such as enoxaparin are only given by injections under the skin. Their dose is somewhat easier to regulate than unfractionated heparin. However, their effectiveness for preventing blood clots in women with the highest risk, such as those with a mechanical heart valve, has not been established.

Overall, using heparin for most of pregnancy is associated with lower direct risk to the baby, but greater risk to the mother—and so, indirectly, to the baby too. This is because heparin is less likely than warfarin to prevent blood clots from forming over the course of the pregnancy. Using warfarin, especially during weeks six to twelve of pregnancy, carries the least risk to the mother but the highest risk to the baby.

There's no one right answer to this problem. Current recommendations include giving mothers with the highest risk of forming blood clots, such as those with older forms of mechanical mitral valves, warfarin throughout the pregnancy—and hoping for the best with the baby. Using lower doses of warfarin may help reduce the baby's risk. Another alternative is to use daily injections of heparin in one of its two forms (fractionated or unfractionated) at the time of peak risk to the baby, during the first twelve weeks of pregnancy. The mother is then switched to warfarin until about two weeks before delivery. At that time, warfarin is stopped and heparin is restarted. Doing this latter switch is routine in any woman taking warfarin. This is because it's easier to reverse the blood thinning effects of heparin than the effects of warfarin and thus reduce the risk of bleeding at the time of birth.

Women at lower risk of blood clots forming during pregnancy, such as those with mechanical aortic valves, have a third alternative. They can use only heparin injections throughout pregnancy and avoid warfarin entirely.

Clearly, if any of these issues on using warfarin during pregnancy apply to you, it's important that you talk with your doctor about the risks and benefits of each of these treatment choices. You can then decide what choice is best for you.

Medications the mother takes can still harm the baby after delivery if she decides to breastfeed. Many heart medications can pass from her bloodstream into breast milk. Some, like digoxin, aspirin, and metoprolol are not considered a significant threat to the baby. Breastfeeding while taking these medications is not prohibited. Interestingly, considering all the problems it can cause during pregnancy, warfarin can be safely used if the mother is breastfeeding her baby. On the other hand, it is recommended that statins and amiodarone should not be used either during pregnancy or with breastfeeding.

Pregnancy and Cardiac Testing

Certain standard heart tests and procedures can cause increased risk to the baby. They can also occasionally carry more than the usual risk to the mother too. At the "safe" end of the scale, an EKG, Holter monitor, or transthoracic echocardiogram carry essentially no risk to the mother or the baby. The very small risk to the mother and baby from doing a transesophageal echocardiogram is mostly due to the small doses of intravenous medications that might be used to make her drowsy before doing the test. The transesophageal echocardiogram itself carries very little risk to either mother or baby.

Exercise stress testing can be safely done, particularly early during pregnancy. However, in the later months of pregnancy, the level of exercise done should be limited to less than the mother's maximum ability to exercise. The baby's heart rate should also be monitored during the test.

Any test that exposes the baby to radiation, such as a chest X-ray, myocardial perfusion imaging, or coronary angiogram, should be avoided if possible. However, if one of these tests is needed, the amount of radiation exposure to both the mother and baby should be kept as low as possible. As we discussed earlier, radiation exposure to the baby early during pregnancy can lead to an increased risk of birth defects. This risk becomes lower later in pregnancy. However, even then radiation exposure can lead to slower growth and possibly development of cancer and leukemia during childhood.

A chest X-ray exposes the baby to only a very small amount of radiation. The amount of radiation exposure to the baby is higher with a nuclear heart scan, but it is still low enough to produce little risk. Tests like coronary angiography that use a fluoroscopy machine have the potential for the greatest radiation exposure. Shielding the mother's abdomen with a lead apron during a test that uses X-rays or fluoroscopy helps minimize the baby's exposure to radiation. Inserting catheters through blood vessels in the arm rather than the leg and avoiding any direct use of the fluoroscope over the abdomen can also help reduce the baby's risk.

Fortunately, most women with heart problems tolerate pregnancy well. Even those with even moderate to severe heart disease can usually be treated with medicines or procedures that minimize the risk to both mother and baby. However, as we've pointed out, there are exceptions to this rule. If you are a woman with heart disease who is pregnant or is thinking about becoming pregnant, it's essential that you talk with your doctor about what your specific risks are and what can be done to reduce them.

Chapter 13 Summary
- ♥ Heart rate normally increases during pregnancy. Blood pressure normally decreases during the first six months of pregnancy, then gradually increases back to near normal.

- ♥ Coronary artery disease, heart failure, heart valve disease, and high blood pressure can generally be treated with medications alone during pregnancy.

- ♥ Mild congenital heart disease in the mother usually does not cause significant risk to her or her baby during pregnancy. Severe congenital heart disease and significant pulmonary hypertension can increase the mother's risk of death and other complications during pregnancy.

- ♥ Heart medications vary in the risk they pose to the baby during pregnancy. Warfarin carries a particularly high risk to the unborn baby.

- ♥ Heart tests that use radiation should be used only if necessary during pregnancy and with steps taken to minimize radiation exposure to both the mother and unborn baby.

Chapter 14: Women and Heart Disease
When a Woman's Heart Breaks

Chapter Preview:

Medications and Menopause
Past and current recommendations on hormone replacement therapy

Birth Control Pills and Heart Disease
Risks of birth control pills

Medicines and Sex in Women
Heart medications and sexual dysfunction in women

Women and Coronary Artery Disease
Differences between men and women in risk and symptoms of heart disease

Evaluating Coronary Artery Disease in Women
Differences between women and men in symptoms of coronary artery disease
Differences between women and men in usefulness of stress tests
Differences between women and men with a heart attack

Treating Coronary Artery Disease in Women
Coronary angioplasty
Coronary artery bypass graft surgery

Women and Stroke
Comparison of stroke in women and men

Women and Arrhythmias
Comparison of types of arrhythmias in women and men

Women and Heart Valve Disease
Mitral valve prolapse and mitral stenosis

Women and Heart Failure
　Comparison of heart failure in women and men
　Medications and heart failure
　Stress cardiomyopathy

ON HER FIRST day of medical school, Maryellen arrived at 7 a.m. sharp, even though the doors to the lecture room didn't open until 8 a.m. She took a seat in the second row. After all, she didn't want to appear overly eager.

Dr. Fred Robbins, dean of Case Western Reserve University School of Medicine, welcomed the first-year class. He was one of the Nobel Prize winners who had helped to lay the groundwork that led to Sabin's and Salk's polio vaccines.

"Half of what we are about to teach you is wrong," Dr. Robbins announced.

"We just don't know what half!"

Although the class laughed, it only took a matter of months to realize that what Dr. Robbins said was no joke!

Medications and Menopause

Dr. Robbins' statement is clearly illustrated by the different viewpoints about estrogen replacement therapy the medical community has put forth over the years. Before menopause, when estrogen levels fall and menstrual periods stop, women have a significantly lower chance of developing coronary artery disease (CAD) compared to men the same age with similar risk factors. Roughly speaking, the risk of CAD in a woman prior to menopause is about the same as a man 10 years younger. Before menopause, estrogen levels are much higher in women than men. The fall in estrogen levels that occurs during and after menopause is associated with a significant increase in the risk of a woman developing CAD.

The "logical" conclusion is that, if estrogen levels are restored to what they were before menopause, the risk of developing CAD would also fall. The fact that estrogen replacement can lower LDL cholesterol, increase HDL cholesterol, and reduce blood sugar—effects that reduce the risk of developing CAD—seemed to support this idea. Some effects of giving estrogen—it increases triglycerides and the risk of developing blood clots—were recognized as being potentially harmful to the heart. However, these bad effects were not thought to be as significant as estrogen's good effects.

Some early studies did, in fact, suggest that estrogen was, overall, beneficial. These studies contributed to the expanded use of estrogen to help prevent heart disease in the 1990s. In general, postmenopausal women were often prescribed a combination of estrogen and another female hormone, progesterone. More than twenty years ago it was found that giving estrogen by itself increased a woman's risk of developing cancer in the lining of her uterus (endometrial cancer) by as much as five times. Giving estrogen and progesterone together—"hormone replacement therapy"—negated this risk. If a woman had a hysterectomy and no longer had a uterus, estrogens might be given alone.

However, over the past several years a series of large studies reached very different conclusions about the effects of hormone replacement therapy on the heart. They showed that using estrogen and progesterone together in postmenopausal women did *not* reduce the risk of heart attack or death from CAD. These hormones weren't beneficial for preventing these problems in postmenopausal women regardless of whether they were known to have heart disease or not. Hormone replacement therapy also did not reduce how rapidly blockages in the coronary arteries worsened.

In fact, some studies found hormone replacement therapy might even *increase* the risk to the heart, especially in the first year after this therapy was started. Based on this research, it's currently recommended that hormone replacement therapy should not be used in postmenopausal women to prevent heart disease.

However, these latest studies still may not be the final word. It may be that a dose of estrogen different from the ones used in these studies *might* be beneficial. It's also possible that estrogen might be useful in *some* women based on their genetics or the age they start taking it. For example, in one large study that showed increased risk to the heart from hormone replacement therapy, the women ranged in age from 50 to 79 years old. The average age was 63. Those women who were between 60 to 69 years old had only a tiny increase in risk of heart attack or death from CAD. On the other hand, those between 70 and 79 years old had the greatest risk. The question of whether a particular group of women might reduce their risk of heart problems by taking hormone replacement therapy is still being studied.

Of course, this whole issue is complicated even more by the fact that hormone replacement therapy can both help and hurt other parts of the body beside the heart. Hormone replacement therapy can increase risk of breast cancer, blood clots in the leg, and stroke. However, this therapy reduces "hot flashes," osteoporosis, and hip fractures. Overall, hormone replacement therapy appears to be a mixed blessing. It can be difficult to determine whether or not its benefits exceed its risks in a particular woman. Once again, however, until more studies are done, hormone replacement therapy should not be given to prevent or treat heart disease.

Stay tuned for further developments on this issue.

A full discussion of the management of menopausal symptoms and the role of hormone replacement therapy is outside the scope of this book. Consult your gynecologist or other primary health care provider for recommendations regarding your particular situation.

Birth Control Pills and Heart Disease
Using estrogens *before* menopause, in the form of birth control pills, is also associated with increased risk to the heart and blood vessels. Estrogens increase the risk of heart attack, blood clots in the legs and lungs, and stroke. This risk is low in healthy women less than 35 years old. However, if a woman smokes or has a previous history of CAD, blood clots, stroke, hypertension, untreated high cholesterol, or diabetes, the risk of using birth control pills increases significantly, especially if she is 35 years old or older. The more of these risk factors a woman has, the higher the risk.

Reducing the risk of taking birth control pills obviously involves decreasing or eliminating these other risk factors as much as possible. As much as she might like to, a woman can't change her age. However, she can stop smoking and take the medicines her doctor prescribes for hypertension, diabetes, and high cholesterol. Once as many risk factors as possible are controlled, she can discuss with her doctor whether or not the overall medical risks of taking birth control pills outweigh their benefits to her.

Medicines and Sex in Women

Although men are more vulnerable to sexual dysfunction caused by cardiac medications, some of these medications can affect women too. As in men, beta-blockers are most notorious for doing this. They can decrease sexual desire in women. Beta-blockers can also cause depression, which may indirectly contribute to loss of interest in sex. Other commonly used heart medications that can decrease sexual desire in women include statins, clonidine, spironolactone, digoxin, and calcium channel blockers. Methyldopa, used for treatment of high blood pressure, can inhibit a woman from having an orgasm.

Medications like silfenadil (Viagra) have a good success rate in treating sexual dysfunction in men. There are anecdotal accounts and "testimonials" that they may help women too. However, so far no good studies have proven that Viagra and similar medications are effective for sexual dysfunction in women. These medications are currently not approved for this use. However, a woman can at least benefit indirectly from these medications based on what the man in her life can now do for her.

Women and Coronary Artery Disease

Women also differ from men in how often certain heart problems occur in them and the way they occur. The relative protection premenopausal women have against developing CAD compared to age-matched men is a major example of this. However, this advantage falls significantly not only after menopause, but also if the premenopausal woman has other risk factors for CAD. For example, a premenopausal woman with diabetes has the same risk of developing CAD as a man who is her age and doesn't have diabetes. A woman with diabetes who has a heart attack is more likely to die from it than a man with diabetes.

High blood pressure is more common before age 55 in men than in women. After age 55, however, more women have high blood pressure than men. In fact, after age 45 about half of women have high blood pressure. Current guidelines for treating high blood pressure are the same for men and women. Previous studies have, in general, shown that medications used to treat high blood pressure are similarly effective in men and women. However, some studies have shown that women may need a greater number of different blood pressure medicines than men to achieve the same level of blood pressure control.

Women can also have high blood pressure occur for reasons that don't affect men. As we discussed in Chapter 13, women can develop high blood pressure during pregnancy as part of preeclampsia or eclampsia. Birth control pills, a medication used only by women (for obvious reasons), can by itself increase blood pressure.

Women generally have better levels of cholesterol than men prior to menopause. However, after menopause cholesterol levels are similar in men and women. In older women, having elevated triglycerides and low HDL cholesterol may carry relatively higher risk than an elevation in the LDL cholesterol. The level of LDL cholesterol may have more significance in men. The statins used to treat high cholesterol appear to have similar effectiveness and benefit in both men and women. However, so far there is not enough information on the benefit in women of other types of cholesterol-lowering medications like gemfibrozil, which primarily lowers triglycerides rather than LDL cholesterol. For unclear reasons, trying to lower cholesterol by reducing fats and calories in the diet seems, on average, to be less effective in women than in men.

Evaluating Coronary Artery Disease in Women
Chest pain and CAD can be more difficult to evaluate in women than in men. Many women, especially younger women, have chest pain that's not typical for angina and is not due to significant blockages in their coronary arteries. Their pain is more likely than men's to be due to heart problems that are less life-threatening and less common than CAD. There may be temporary spasm of a coronary artery, reducing blood supply to the heart until the spasm goes away. The coronary arteries may not relax enough to increase blood flow to the heart when it's needed ("impaired vasodilatory reserve"). Mitral valve prolapse, an abnormality seen in young women, can also cause chest pain.

Women are also more likely than men to have chest pain that isn't caused by the heart. These other causes include pain coming from the bones or muscles of the chest, the lungs, and problems with the stomach and esophagus.

On the other hand, if a woman really does have CAD, it may be more difficult to recognize it. This is because her chest pain is more likely to have features that aren't "classic" for angina. Instead of having angina primarily with exertion, women are more likely than men to have angina when under stress or during sleep. Their pain is also less likely to be described as a "pressure."

A premenopausal woman is more likely than a man her age to have a "false-positive" exercise stress test. This means the electrocardiogram (EKG) shows evidence of the heart not getting enough blood due to

CAD, even though the woman really *doesn't* have CAD. A false-positive test is thought to be due largely to the effects of estrogen on the EKG. Adding an imaging test, such as an echocardiogram or a myocardial perfusion imaging (nuclear) study, to the stress test improves its reliability. However, if the EKG part of the stress test *doesn't* show any changes to suggest the heart isn't getting enough blood, this normal result is more reliable for excluding CAD in a woman than in a man. Men have a higher chance of really having CAD even though the EKG part of the test doesn't detect it ("false-negative" test).

Bigger problems occur when a woman has a heart attack. Women are more likely than men to have a "silent" heart attack—one that either doesn't cause symptoms or causes symptoms that aren't recognized as being due to a heart attack. Women are less likely to have the prolonged, crushing pain beneath the breastbone that's "classic" for a heart attack. Instead, they are more likely to have less clear-cut symptoms like pain in the jaw, neck, or belly, as well as nausea and palpitations.

If a woman with a heart attack makes it to the hospital, she is more likely than a man her age to have complications such as heart failure, stroke, and death. In fact, younger women have about twice the chance of dying in the hospital from their heart attack than men their same age. Even if they make it out of the hospital, these younger women have a death rate higher than their male counterparts for as long as three years after the heart attack.

Treating Coronary Artery Disease in Women

Men and women with CAD have roughly similar initial success rates when their disease is treated with angioplasty. However, women have a higher rate of complications with the procedure. These complications include bleeding, sudden clotting off the coronary artery blockage treated with angioplasty, and death. The difference in outcomes between men and women is even greater with coronary artery bypass graft surgery (CABG). Women are more likely to die in the hospital after the procedure than men who are their same age. Young women in particular are more likely to die after CABG when compared to young men of the same age. Other serious complications such as heart attack, stroke, and bleeding are also more likely to occur in women than in men. If they make it out of the hospital, women are less likely to be free of angina and to return to work than men. These women also have more overall disability than men. However, women who make it out of the hospital after CABG don't have any greater chance of dying, having a heart attack, or needing a second CABG in the future than men.

Why women do worse than men in many ways with these procedures is still debated. Many women have smaller bodies than men, and their coronary arteries are often smaller and harder to work on than a man's. Factors such as a higher incidence of diabetes and hypertension in women may also be involved. However, a final answer is still being sought.

Women and Stroke

Men and women have, overall, a roughly equal rate of having peripheral arterial disease and stroke. Stroke is more likely to be caused by blockages in the carotid (neck) arteries in men, while in women it's more likely due to blood clots going to the brain. Women also tend to be older than men when they have their first stroke.

Women and Arrhythmias

Certain types of abnormal heart rhythms (arrhythmias) are more likely to occur in women than in men. "Inappropriate sinus tachycardia" occurs when a person's normal heart rhythm is abnormally fast. It is more likely to occur in women than men. One arrhythmia that causes fast heart rates, paroxysmal supraventricular tachycardia, is somewhat more common in women than men. On the other hand, another arrhythmia that can make the heart go too fast, atrial fibrillation, is more likely to occur in men.

Serious arrhythmias originating in the lower chambers (ventricles) of the heart, such as ventricular tachycardia, are somewhat more common in men than in women. The risk of dying from one of these ventricular arrhythmias is also greater in men.

Women and Heart Valve Disease

Mitral valve prolapse, an abnormality in the way the mitral valve closes, is more common in women than men. However, men are more likely to have serious complications from mitral valve prolapse, like the valve becoming infected or leaking so severely it might require surgery. Mitral stenosis, a narrowing of the mitral valve caused by rheumatic fever, is more common in women. However, damage to the aortic valve due to rheumatic fever is more frequent in men.

Women and Heart Failure

Heart failure tends to occur at a later age in women than in men. However, it's more common in elderly women than in elderly men. In women, heart failure is more likely to be associated with hypertension and diabetes. On the other hand, men are more likely to have heart failure caused by an old heart attack.

The effectiveness of most kinds of medical treatment for heart failure seems similar in men and women. However, some major studies using angiotensin-converting enzyme (ACE) inhibitors either included only a relatively small number of women, or the studies suggested that men might respond somewhat better to ACE inhibitors than women did. One study using digoxin even showed that women taking it for heart failure had a higher risk of dying than men who received it. This increased risk was found, however, to be associated with higher levels of digoxin in the bloodstream. Women taking a dose small enough to produce lower blood levels did not have increased risk of death from digoxin and the medicine was helpful in them.

Can loss of a loved one or other emotional stress really cause a woman's heart to "break"? Recent reports indicate this actually does happen. Emotional stress can temporarily "stun" the heart, causing chest pain, changes on the EKG, and even abnormal blood test results indicating damage to the heart that mimic a heart attack. This "stress cardiomyopathy" has been reported predominantly in women, after events such as the death of a spouse, parent, or child. For example, in a report published in the February 10, 2005 issue of the *New England Journal of Medicine*, 18 of the 19 patients found to have this problem were women.

Unlike the usual patient with a heart attack, coronary angiography done in patients with stress cardiomyopathy typically shows no significant blockage in the arteries of the heart. However, heart function is significantly and often severely reduced, and these individuals can have shortness of breath and other evidence of heart failure. The left ventricle shows a characteristic shape and pattern of abnormal motion on echocardiography and with cardiac catheterization (the injection of contrast—"dye"—into the left ventricle when coronary angiography is done). The part of the left ventricle near the mitral valve—the "base" of the left ventricle—typically contracts normally. However, the rest of the left ventricle contracts poorly, particularly its far end or "apex," and appears to "bulge" or "balloon" out. This makes the left ventricle look somewhat like a jar with a narrow neck.

Because of this appearance, stress cardiomyopathy is also called "transient left ventricular apical ballooning" or "takotsubo cardiomyopathy." The latter name is given because the left ventricle resembles a "takotsubo"—a fishing pot with a narrow neck and wide base used in Japan to trap an octopus—and initial descriptions of this problem were reported in Japan. Stress cardiomyopathy may be caused by spasm of the coronary arteries, temporarily reducing blood supply to the heart, and possibly by direct damage to the heart caused by excessive catecholamines—chemicals like adrenaline, or "epinephrine"—produced by stress. Fortunately, heart function typically returns to normal within days to weeks. Most women and men recover completely from their stress cardiomyopathy.

Overall, the lesson to be learned from what we've discussed in this chapter is this: while men and women are similar in many ways, as in other areas of life, when it comes to heart disease, there are just enough differences between them to make things interesting!

Chapter 14 Summary

♥ Hormone replacement therapy is now not generally recommended to help prevent coronary artery disease in postmenopausal women.

♥ Birth control pills are associated with increased risk of heart attack, blood clots, stroke, and other problems in women, particularly if they have certain risk factors. These risk factors include an age of 35 years or older, smoking, diabetes, and high blood pressure.

♥ Some heart medications, including beta-blockers, can cause sexual dysfunction in women.

♥ Women with coronary artery disease can be more difficult to identify than men with coronary artery disease based on their symptoms and results of stress tests.

♥ Women have a higher risk of death and some other complications than men following heart attack, coronary angioplasty, or coronary artery bypass graft surgery.

Chapter 15: Your Lifestyle and Your Love Life
Health Choices That Affect Your Sex Life

Chapter Preview:
Diet and Heart Disease
    Recommended types of foods
    Recommendations for fats, proteins, and carbohydrates
Weight Loss
    Body mass index and target range for weight
    Risk of death and other health problems in the overweight and obese
    Guidelines for losing weight
Exercise
    Targets for performing exercise
    Benefits of exercise
Nutritional Supplements
    Comparison to conventional medications
    Limitations of nutritional supplements
Heart Disease and Alcohol
    Benefits and risks
Tobacco and the Heart
    Risks of tobacco use
    Risks of passive smoking
    Methods to help quit smoking
Illegal Drugs
    Cocaine
    Other illegal drugs
Health and Sex
    How a healthy lifestyle helps your sex life
Sex and Alcohol
    Sexual dysfunction and alcohol use
Sex and Tobacco
    Sexual dysfunction and tobacco use

Heart Disease and Sexually Transmitted Diseases
Syphilis and gonorrhea
Acquired immune deficiency syndrome (AIDS)

THERE ARE SOME heart problems that occur for reasons outside a person's control, like their age, genetics, or just bad luck. However, the odds of developing atherosclerosis—the underlying process that causes coronary artery disease (CAD) and blockages in other arteries in the body—can be significantly reduced by what you can do. Even if a person has already developed a cardiac problem, living a healthy lifestyle can improve both your quantity and quality of life—including your sex life.

The patients Henry sees as a cardiologist cover a very broad range as to how motivated they are to participate in their own care. At one end of the spectrum are the "enthusiasts"—people who radically altered how they live after a heart attack. They are the ones who faithfully go to the cardiac rehabilitation program for counseling and exercise, eat a prudent diet, and have discarded their cigarettes. Their office visits are a bit longer than average due to the meticulously detailed logs they bring in for review containing daily measurements of their blood pressure, heart rate, and weight. They also typically ask many questions about what they can do to keep in good shape. Some are reluctant to take medications and prefer natural treatments like diet and exercise to keep healthy. However, they do take the medicines that are needed to reduce their risk of further heart problems as much as possible.

At the other end of the scale are the "Why did you even bother to come to see me?" patients. Their telltale signs might include the open pack of cigarettes in the shirt pocket and nonchalant look when they are asked if they've been taking all their medications. "Oh, I never got that one filled," or "I ran out of it two months ago," are common responses. Those patients that do (sometimes) take their medicines use them as magical antidotes. As Henry tells them, taking a cholesterol-lowering pill and then chowing down on a couple of quarter pound hamburgers and handfuls of fries is like spraying water on a fire with one hand and pouring gasoline on it with the other! Their idea of an exercise program is pressing the buttons on the TV remote as often as possible. Needless to say, cardiologists are more likely to see these patients again in the hospital rather than in the office—or end up sending a sympathy card to their surviving family members.

Most people, of course, fall between these two extremes. Maybe you're one of them yourself. After you leave your doctor's office, what can *you* do to improve your health?

Diet and Heart Disease
Maryellen grew up in an ethnic family that centered its activities around good food. She has struggled with weight problems for most of her life and consequently has a great deal of sympathy for people trying to follow a healthy diet. She classifies herself as a food addict. She has hidden brownies in the bathroom and scavenged through the trash looking for sweets.

Eating a healthy diet is good for both the heart and the rest of the body. But what exactly is a healthy diet? This is actually a complicated topic, with many types of diets being promoted to the general public and to specific groups such as heart patients and diabetics.

For heart patients, some of the types of diets that have been suggested include the "Mediterranean-style," the "Prudent Diet," and the "Heart Healthy" diet. Large medical organizations like the American Heart Association (www.americanheart.org) have also issued guidelines regarding diet. Although the details vary, all of these "standard" diets share certain basic recommendations. They suggest that, if a person is already at a good weight for one's age, height, and sex, the total number of calories he or she eats in a day should be just enough to keep him or her at a good weight. If a person is obese, the number of calories he or she eats per day should be just enough to cause a safe rate of weight loss until the "ideal" weight is reached. Foods that are protective against developing or worsening atherosclerosis are encouraged. Foods that increase cholesterol and weight are discouraged.

Eating at least five portions of fruits and vegetables per day is a common recommendation in these diets. These foods contain fiber, antioxidants like vitamin C, and other natural nutrients. They have been shown to reduce the risk of developing CAD and of dying from it.

Foods with whole grains like wheat, corn, and oats also contain vitamins and minerals the body needs. These grains also reduce the risk of CAD. However, they also contain starches and sugar that may disproportionately increase blood sugar and triglycerides—*not* a good thing. Eating at least two to three portions of whole-grain foods per day is recommended as a good balance between these effects. The type of grain-containing food eaten also makes a difference. Whole-grain foods like whole wheat bread are better than those containing refined grains, such as white bread or other foods made from white flour. Foods high in starches, like bread or pasta, are considered better than those high in sugar.

Legumes are plants that include beans, peas, and soybeans. The evidence that eating them reduces risk of developing CAD is not as strong as for fruits, other vegetables, and grains. However, there is enough evidence to recommend legumes as part of a healthy diet. Nuts, particularly walnuts and almonds, have also been found to be beneficial. In several studies, people who ate nuts more than four times a week had a significantly lower risk of developing CAD or having a heart attack than those who ate them once a week or less. However, it's doubtful that eating nuts when they're embedded in a king-size candy bar has an overall beneficial effect.

Fish and fish oil contain nutrients like omega-3 fatty acids that lower triglycerides and have other beneficial effects. The American Heart Association recommends eating two servings of fish every week. Fatty fish like mackerel, salmon, and sardines are preferred. Although not thought to be as beneficial as getting it from eating fish, capsules containing omega-3 fatty acids can also be taken. The suggested amount is up to one gram per day, or up to three to four grams per day if recommended by a doctor to lower high triglycerides.

Although several popular diets offer a different opinion, conventional wisdom is that foods high in certain fats and cholesterol should be restricted. Saturated fatty acids are present in meats, dairy products, and tropical oils like coconut oil and palm oil. They raise LDL ("bad") cholesterol. Polyunsaturated fatty acids, like those in olive oil, corn oil, safflower oil, and canola oil, don't increase LDL cholesterol and are preferred.

Trans fatty acids are produced when polyunsaturated fatty acids are "hydrogenated" to keep them from spoiling. They are present in foods labeled as containing "partially hydrogenated vegetable oils." These include margarine, especially stick margarine, and many baked goods high in fat content, like cakes and cookies—Maryellen's favorite foods! *Trans* fatty acids raise LDL cholesterol and can also lower HDL ("good") cholesterol.

In recommendations made in July 2006, the American Heart Association suggests that the general population should limit total cholesterol intake to 300 mg per day. People with heart disease or at risk for developing heart disease should take in only 200 mg per day of cholesterol. Eating lean meats and more white meat like chicken rather than red meat like beef is generally recommended.

The total amount of fat in a person's diet is recommended to be 25% to 35% of the total calories eaten in a day. Most of this fat should be in the form of polyunsaturated fatty acids. Saturated fatty acids should be less than 7% of total calories eaten every day. *Trans* fatty acids should be less than 1% of total calories. The remaining calories should be split between proteins and carbohydrates, with a mildly greater percentage of the latter being favored. It's also important to know when planning your diet and calculating the total number of calories you eat in a day that fats contain 9 calories per gram, while proteins and carbohydrates contain only 4 calories per gram.

Several "low-carb" diets have also been proposed specifically to enhance weight loss. Comparisons between diets low in carbohydrates and more conventional ones low in fat show that both can lead to significant weight loss. However, weight loss is usually faster with a low-carbohydrate diet. Low-fat diets can decrease LDL cholesterol and triglycerides while raising HDL cholesterol. These are all good effects. However, while low-carbohydrate diets lower triglycerides and raise HDL cholesterol, they cause little change in LDL cholesterol. There is also some concern that, because low-carbohydrate diets downplay eating fruits, vegetables, and whole-grain foods and favor the use of more foods with saturated fat and *trans* fat, in the long run these diets could increase the risk of atherosclerosis. However, as of this writing the overall relative risks and benefits of low-carbohydrate and low-fat diets have yet to be established.

The DASH (Dietary Approaches to Stop Hypertension) diet is particularly useful in patients with high blood pressure. It emphasizes reduction of salt (sodium chloride) in the diet and includes foods rich in potassium, magnesium, and calcium. As with low-fat diets, the DASH diet encourages the eating of fruits, vegetables, and whole-grain foods, as well as low-fat dairy products. Restricting salt intake is also very important in patients with weakened heart function and heart failure to avoid excess water retention. The current general recommendation for salt intake is to limit it to no more than 2.3 grams of sodium per day. This is about 6 grams of salt—around one teaspoonful. People with heart failure and hypertension should try to limit sodium intake to 2 grams per day or less. More information about this diet is located at the website of the National Heart, Lung, and Blood Institute: (www.nhlbi.nih.gov/health/public/heart/hbp/dash/introduction.html).

Weight Loss

Besides improving cholesterol and reducing high blood pressure, it's also important for you to maintain a healthy weight. Being at or close to your recommended weight will not only help you be more active, but it can even help you live longer and also improve your sex life. It may allow you to assume different positions during sex that are not achievable if you are very overweight. If you are obese, losing weight can also increase depth of penile penetration, although it should be noted that the overall length and size of the penis does not necessarily correlate with sexual satisfaction.

The current guidelines for what is a healthy weight are based on the body mass index (BMI). The BMI is just your weight (in kilograms) divided by your height (in meters) squared. If you're uncomfortable using kilograms and meters, take your weight in pounds, divide it by the square of your height in inches, and multiply the result by 703.

The normal range for BMI in adults is 18.5 to 24.9. A man or woman with a BMI of 25 to less than 30 is considered "overweight." A BMI of 30 to less than 40 indicates a person is "obese," while a BMI of 40 or greater means he or she is "extremely" or "morbidly" obese.

For example, a person 6 feet 2 inches (74 inches) tall and weighing 180 pounds has a BMI of about 23.16, which is normal. (A good thing too, since the person we're describing is Henry, the cardiologist part of our writing duo!) You can calculate your own BMI using simple tables and calculators found on an Internet search for "body mass index," or by using the formulas above on your own calculator.

A large study in the *New England Journal of Medicine* (August 24, 2006 issue) showed how being obese or even just overweight significantly increases your risk of dying. In this study, over 500,000 Americans between the ages of 50 to 71 were followed for over 10 years. Men and women with a normal BMI between 23.5 and 24.9 had the lowest risk of death over those 10 years. However, individuals who were overweight (BMI 25 to 29.9) had a 20 to 40% higher risk of death than those with a BMI of 23.5 and 24.9. The risk of death was even greater in people who were obese, with a BMI of 30 or more, and increased steadily as BMI rose. Obese people had a risk of dying that was two to at least three times higher than those with a normal BMI of 23.5 to 24.9. These results applied to both men and women and to all racial and ethnic groups.

For people who are overweight or obese, not all fat is created equal. "Truncal" or "apple-shaped" obesity—accumulation of excess fat mainly around the belly—is more common in men. It is associated with increased risk of developing heart disease, particularly CAD. "Peripheral" or "pear-shaped" obesity—more common in women, with fat deposited mainly in the buttocks and hips—is not associated with increased risk of heart disease by itself. However, all types of obesity increase a person's risk of developing or worsening diabetes, high blood pressure, and other health problems.

Losing weight is partly a matter of physics. In general, if you burn more calories than you eat, you'll lose weight. If you burn fewer calories than you eat, you'll gain weight. To lose weight at a healthy rate, the American Heart Association guidelines suggest that you eat 500 to 1000 calories less than you burn each day. Since you have to go 3500 calories on the "negative" side to lose one pound, this works out to a target of losing 1 to 2 pounds per week. The rule of thumb to determine about how many calories you burn in a day is to multiply your weight (in pounds) by 15 if you're moderately active, or by 13 if you're not. Subtract 500 or 1000 from that number and you have your maximum calorie target for the day to lose weight at a healthy pace. Once again, the "value" of the calories you take in is also important. Getting 100 calories from an apple is healthier than getting those 100 calories from a cookie, and it really does help keep the doctor away.

Certain medical conditions such as an underactive thyroid gland (hypothyroidism) or diabetes can make weight loss difficult. Psychological factors such as depression, anxiety, and anger may also make it difficult for some people to achieve and maintain a healthy body weight. These individuals may use overeating as a means to cope with stress. Consulting your physician and/or a mental health professional may be helpful to explore these possibilities. Your health care provider may also refer you to a dietitian who can give you individualized advice on losing weight.

It may also help you to join a weight-loss support group. When we lived in St. Louis, Maryellen belonged to Weight Watchers. At our current home in the Ozarks, Maryellen is a member of TOPS (Take Off Pounds Sensibly). The encouragement and experiences she shares with others help inspire her to stick with her weight-loss goals.

Exercise
Besides eating right, performing regular exercise is also important to help you lose weight and to keep from

regaining it once you've reached your target weight. No, that doesn't mean working out at the gym until your physique looks like Arnold Schwartzenegger in his prime. Only a few of us have the genes for that, and we may also be a little too old to become belated body builders. Also, lifting *heavy* weights is not a good idea for people with heart disease. This type of "isometric" exercise causes a higher and faster elevation in blood pressure than "isotonic" (aerobic) exercise like walking and puts more strain on the heart. Light weightlifting is safe and helpful for the majority of people. Many can also safely do moderate weightlifting. Check with your doctor to see what level of weightlifting is reasonably safe for you.

Current guidelines for healthy adults and those who have stable, controlled heart problems include performing moderate levels of exercise, like brisk walking or calisthenics, for at least 30 minutes on most days of the week. For people who've had a previous heart attack, the target is to exercise 30 to 60 minutes every day of the week. If this exercise can't be done all at once—for example, while taking a long walk—you can break it down into smaller blocks, such as 10 minute each, to get that total of 30 minutes or more. "Exercise" can also mean light sports like playing a quick game of golf (preferably not using a cart) or badminton, being physically active as part of your job, doing work around the house, etc. If you have been very inactive, it's better to start out below these targets and work up to them.

Maryellen belongs to Curves, a popular exercise franchise designed for women. Although she doesn't look forward to exercising itself, she does look forward to seeing the many friends she's made there, which motivates her to "stick with the program."

If someone who's previously not been exercising suddenly decides to take up really vigorous exercise like jogging, tennis, or cycling in the Tour de France, this person should check with his or her doctor first. While most heart attacks and serious arrhythmias occur when a person is resting, asleep, or doing only light activity, they can occasionally occur when a person is doing something strenuous. Although the need for doing this is still controversial, it's been suggested that "healthy" men age 45 and older and women age 55 and older may have an exercise stress test done before starting a vigorous exercise program. The stress test is used to screen for evidence of heart disease, especially CAD, and to see how healthy a person really is, before finding out the hard way he or she isn't.

The benefits of exercise include helping a person get to and maintain a healthy weight, conditioning the body's muscles to be more efficient (and so require the heart to work less), improving control of blood sugar in diabetics, and lowering blood pressure. And, of course, it can improve your quality of life by making you feel better and able to do more than you could before —including having sex with your spouse!

Nutritional Supplements
There are a bewildering variety of nutritional (dietary) supplements available for people to take at their own discretion. Some contain nutrients, like vitamins C or E, or amino acids like arginine that are found in foods but concentrated at a high dose in the form of a pill. Others contain "natural" ingredients like herbs and other plants, such as garlic, green tea, cayenne, ginseng, and so on.

It's been suggested that some of these preparations can be effective for lowering blood pressure and cholesterol, as well as helping diabetes and other health problems. Evidence that they actually do this is, overall, mild. The use of many of these substances is based on traditional, "home remedies" that predate the availability of modern medications. Only a very small number of these supplements have been studied for their effectiveness and safety with the rigorous standards used for conventional medicines.

For example, results of studies using vitamin E supplements to either prevent heart problems in healthy individuals or people who have had a heart attack have been inconsistent, with some reporting a mild benefit while others showed no benefit or even a mild degree of harm. On the other hand, omega-3 fatty acid pills have been found to lower triglycerides in appropriate doses. Red yeast rice extract contains substances with chemical activity similar to statins (like lovastatin) and can also reduce cholesterol. Garlic may, at least temporarily, lower cholesterol.

Speaking of garlic, Maryellen fondly recalls Henry's first meeting with her parents. Her mother asked him if she could suck on peppermint candy to treat chest pain. He told her he wasn't sure if it would really help her heart, but if she ever needed to have CPR (cardiopulmonary resuscitation) at least she would have nice breath for the person doing the mouth-to-mouth resuscitation on her. Because of his diplomatic response, her parents approved of him as their future son-in-law. (Besides, everyone wants his or her daughter to marry a cardiologist!)

Some of Henry's patients are very enthusiastic about taking nutritional supplements. It's not unusual for the number they're taking to be several times greater than the number of medicines he's prescribed for them. However, for the vast majority of these nutritional supplements, there's no convincing evidence one way or the other whether they are really beneficial are not and what their potential risks are.

Another risk is that, since the manufacture of these supplements is not as tightly regulated as conventional medications are, there's less certainty that you're really getting what it says on the label. Even if it contains the right substance, the actual amount of it (especially with herbal and similar preparations) may vary widely from manufacturer to manufacturer, if for no other reason than differences in how the herb or other plant material is processed.

Certain nutritional supplements also interfere with the actions of some standard medications. For example, St. John's wort—used as a treatment for mild to moderate depression—reduces the effectiveness of many medications, including some used for heart disease such as verapamil and digoxin. And, as with conventional medications, side effects can also occur with some of these supplements. For example, in 2004 the Food and Drug Administration banned the sale of preparations containing ephedra, a substance used for weight loss and found in a number of plants, following reports that it had caused serious harm. Ephedra was found to significantly increase heart rate and blood pressure in some individuals, and it increased the risk of heart attack and stroke.

In short, if you are thinking about taking nutritional supplements, check with your doctor first regarding both the possible benefits and risks associated with a particular kind. For those naturally found in foods, such as vitamins and omega-3 fatty acids, it's currently recommended that a person should preferably get them from eating foods containing them rather than taking these substances in pill form.

Heart Disease and Alcohol

Alcohol, taken in moderate amounts and particularly in the form of red wine, has been shown to decrease the risk of CAD. This is thought to be at least partly due to it causing an increase in HDL ("good") cholesterol. Current recommendations are that, for adults who already use alcohol, men may have up to two drinks per day. For example, one drink might be a twelve-ounce can of beer or the equivalent amount of alcohol in wine, and so on. Women may have up to one drink per day. This lower recommended amount of alcohol in women is at least partly due to their risk of developing alcohol-related breast cancer.

Of course, too much alcohol is a bad thing from the standpoint of both the heart and the rest of the body. Even the net effect of this "recommended" level of alcohol consumption on a person's overall health is controversial. People with certain health problems like liver disease, a family history of alcoholism, and pregnant women should clearly avoid using alcohol. The "don't drink and drive" rule applies to everyone. So if alcohol isn't part of your usual diet, don't think you *have* to start using it to maintain good heart health. There are other ways of doing it, including eating the kinds and amounts of healthy foods we've discussed previously.

Tobacco and the Heart

While modern Americans often don't eat the healthiest amounts or types of food, each of us needs to eat at least a certain amount to provide his or her body with the nutrients it needs. On the other hand, cigarettes and other tobacco products have no nutritional value at all. Whatever social or psychological benefits a smoker thinks are derived from cigarettes, cigars, or using a pipe, looked at simply from a medical standpoint they are just no darn good. Nearly 500,000 Americans die each year from tobacco-related illnesses. Smoking is a major risk factor for CAD and peripheral arterial disease, especially in people with other risk factors like diabetes and hypertension. Smoking also increases the risk of stroke, particularly in young women taking birth control pills. It has its most disabling and deadly effects on the lungs, causing bronchitis, emphysema, and cancer. Pipes, cigars, and especially chewing tobacco cause cancer in the mouth and throat.

The situation is even more complicated than this. Nonsmokers can be significantly affected by "passive" or "second-hand" smoking—being in the same home, vehicle, or workplace where someone else is smoking. It is even thought that the kind of smoke that nonsmokers inhale by being with a smoker—so-called "sidestream" smoke, coming from the burning tip of the cigarette—is actually more harmful than the "mainstream" smoke inhaled by the smoker.

Studies have shown that the overall risk of an adult nonsmoker developing heart disease, especially CAD, is significantly higher if they are routinely exposed to tobacco smoke. These nonsmokers also have a higher rate of lung problems like asthma, bronchitis, and pneumonia. Children living in a home with a smoker are particularly vulnerable to developing these problems, as well as increasing their risk of developing certain cancers, like leukemia. Passive smoking can also potentially cause a miscarriage in a pregnant woman.

The obvious way to deal with all of these problems is to not start smoking. If you are a smoker, stop. Occasionally Henry has patients who tell him they just decided one day to stop smoking and went "cold turkey." This is usually after they've had a heart attack or received some other bad news about their health. Some of them succeed in staying "former smokers." Unfortunately, most relapse after a while. For the vast majority of smokers, tobacco isn't a choice but an addiction.

One example Henry remembers from many years ago is a man who, right after his coronary angiogram showed he had very severe CAD, demanded to get off the catheterization table and go out for a smoke. He's also had smokers admitted to the hospital with heart attacks who became furious when told they couldn't smoke in the intensive care unit. Before a nurse could stop him, one patient even ripped off the electrode patches on his chest connecting him to a monitor, disconnected the tubing from his intravenous line, and stomped off to the smoking area outside the hospital—in the middle of a snowstorm, trailing blood dripping from his open intravenous line.

A wide variety of methods can be used to help smokers break their habit. One option is participation is a formal smoking cessation program. Techniques used to help smokers include relatively simple methods, such as having their family and friends encourage them to stop smoking, or by teaching relaxation techniques to the smoker. Hypnosis and acupuncture have also been suggested as methods to help reduce tobacco use. Having the smoker "taper" how many cigarettes are smoked each day can be helpful in very heavy smokers—going from four packs per day to one per day certainly can't hurt. However, getting a smoker to cut down at all can be difficult. Also, the individual might compensate for smoking fewer cigarettes by puffing longer and harder on those that are smoked each day, reducing the benefit from cutting back on the total number of cigarettes used.

Using nicotine in the form of a patch, gum, lozenge, nasal spray, or inhaler as a substitute for a cigarette at least represents a step in the right direction. This assumes that the smoker will use it *instead* of a cigarette, rather than with it. A person should not smoke while using a nicotine substitute. The goal is to have the smoker gradually decrease the dose of the nicotine substitute over a period of about several months until, hopefully, the person no longer needs it. The success rate of this method is not high, but it does succeed in some people and can be worth trying.

The only other medication approved by the Food and Drug Administration for smoking cessation besides nicotine substitutes is bupropion (Welbutrin). This medication is also prescribed as an antidepressant. Bupropion can be used with or without a nicotine substitute to help a smoker reduce and, hopefully, stop smoking. Unlike nicotine substitutes, bupropion can be used while the smoker continues to smoke.

Illegal Drugs

Certain illegal drugs can cause serious damage to the heart—and, of course, to the rest of the body. Cocaine is particularly notorious for this. This drug increases heart rate, blood pressure, and how forcefully the heart contracts. These effects increase how much work the heart has to do. Cocaine also decreases the amount of blood the heart gets by causing spasm—temporary narrowing—of the coronary arteries. Less blood is able to get through these "clamped down" arteries. This combination of increased work for the heart and decreased blood supply can be so severe that even people with normal coronary arteries may not get enough blood to their heart and can have a heart attack.

It's no surprise that cocaine is even more dangerous in people who have CAD. Besides its other bad effects on the heart, cocaine also increases the chance of forming blood clots. As we've talked about in earlier chapters, a heart attack is usually caused by a blood clot forming on an atherosclerotic plaque in a coronary artery. Cocaine can make a blood clot form on one of these plaques and cause a heart attack. Long-term use of cocaine increases the risk of developing CAD.

The risk of having a heart attack is greatest within the first hour after using cocaine. Even a small dose of it can cause a heart attack. The risk of heart attack is about the same no matter how the cocaine is used—injected into a vein, smoked ("crack" cocaine), inhaled, etc. Cocaine can also damage the heart without causing an actual heart attack. Long-term use of the drug may cause a cardiomyopathy—an overall weakening of heart function. Even a single use of cocaine can make heart function worsen significantly, although it may recover later.

Cocaine can also cause serious, potentially fatal abnormal heart rhythms. They can occur when the drug makes the heart not get enough blood or causes a heart attack. Cocaine can also cause a life-threatening aortic dissection—a tearing of that large artery's inner lining. This may be due to the drug making a person's blood pressure become dangerously high.

The risks of using cocaine are even greater when it is used with tobacco or alcohol. Heart rate and blood pressure go higher and spasm of the coronary arteries is even worse when a person uses cocaine and smokes cigarettes together. Drinking alcohol when using cocaine can make even a low dose of cocaine more potent.

Abuse of amphetamines ("meth," "speed," "ice") can cause bad effects on the heart similar to cocaine. These drugs also increase heart rate, blood pressure, and cause spasm of the coronary arteries. Like cocaine, amphetamines can cause heart attacks, serious abnormal heart rhythms, and permanent damage to the heart.

Cocaine, amphetamines, heroin, and other illegal drugs can be injected into a vein using a syringe and needle. Using a needle that isn't clean, especially one shared with another illegal drug user, can cause diseases like hepatitis—a viral infection of the liver—and acquired immune deficiency syndrome (AIDS). It can also cause infections on heart valves—infective endocarditis. As we talked about in Chapter 6, the valves on the left side of the heart, the mitral and aortic valves, are much more likely to develop endocarditis than the ones on the right side of the heart, the tricuspid and pulmonic valves. Endocarditis caused by drug abuse is still most likely to involve the mitral and aortic valves. However, endocarditis is significantly more likely to involve the tricuspid and pulmonic valves when this infection is caused by drug abuse than by other problems. Cocaine is reported to have a greater chance of causing endocarditis than using other illegal drugs injected into a vein.

Health and Sex

The relationship of all this preventive medicine to sex is indirect but extremely important. Keeping your body healthy and reducing your risk of heart problems can improve both the quality and quantity of your life. A person who's significantly overweight, very sedentary and poorly conditioned, or who uses tobacco or too much alcohol is also going to be in poor shape for having and enjoying sex. The mechanics of sex become physically difficult. Having intercourse in some positions, especially the more exotic ones, also becomes impossible.

Although the amount of energy needed to have intercourse is only mild to moderate, even this level can be too much for people who don't get enough exercise or who are short of breath due to their smoking. One "workaround" for this is that, if one partner is more physically conditioned than the other, the person in better physical condition can assume the more active sexual position. For example, the woman can get "on top" if her husband gets fatigued easily or if he weighs considerably more than her. However, the best solution is for both partners to get in as good a physical shape as they can. If, after sex, you feel like you've just run the Boston Marathon, it's time to get in better shape!

Sex and Alcohol

Excessive alcohol use can, in the short run, encourage unsafe sex by reducing inhibitions. Alcohol impairs a person's ability to judge the consequences of having sex in a particular situation. Besides this, while intoxicated both men and women are more likely to experience sexual dysfunction. This can include temporary erectile dysfunction (ED) in a man and difficulty achieving orgasm in a woman. Chronic excessive alcohol use can also decrease sexual interest in both men and women. It can even cause a man's testes to atrophy (shrink), contributing to long-term ED.

Sex and Tobacco

Although there are many other reasons to stop smoking, tobacco use increases the chance of a man developing ED by as much as 50%. One proposed reason for this is that nicotine constricts (narrows) arteries, including those in the penis, and limits the amount of blood that can enter the penis to achieve an erection. Just as it does with the coronary arteries, tobacco use also increases the risk of developing atherosclerotic blockages in the arteries to the penis and testes. This reduces blood flow to them. Both this effect and others are associated with production of fewer and more abnormal sperm cells. The risk of developing ED is even greater in male smokers who also have other health problems, like CAD, diabetes, and hypertension.

These problems with men who smoke can obviously affect women indirectly, by increasing the odds of a bedroom failure. Though the effects are not as dramatic as they are in men, women who smoke can also experience sexual dysfunction. Problems with constriction and blockages to the arteries that supply blood to their genitals can lead to decreased arousal and decreased intensity of orgasm.

When we walk into a room to see a patient, we often can tell if the person is a smoker just by looking at him or her. Smokers frequently look older than their age. They typically have more wrinkles on their face and get them earlier than other people their age. This is at least partly due to the fact that nicotine constricts the blood vessels of the face and neck. While all of us eventually look older as we age, smoking can interfere with your love life by making this happen sooner than it has to occur. The odor of smoke on a person's clothing and the effect of tobacco on a person's breath may also be a turnoff to a spouse or potential lover. In short, smoking just doesn't go along with good health or sex.

Heart Disease and Sexually Transmitted Diseases
Maryellen had a very astute dermatologist, "Dr. Stuart," as one of her teachers during medical school. The fascinating thing about Dr. Stuart was that he was blind. Although a brain tumor had cruelly robbed him of his eyesight, his mind was sharp as a scalpel, and he had a wealth of clinical experience to share with medical students. The students would first interview and examine the patients, then step into a conference room to present their findings to Dr. Stuart.

One of Maryellen's patients had an extensive painful-looking rash. He said that the rash started after he ate a fish that he had caught in Lake Erie.

"That fish was a red herring," said Dr. Stuart.

Maryellen had lived in Cleveland all her life, wasn't a fisherman, and had never heard of anyone catching a red herring there. She didn't understand until Dr. Stuart continued.

"That rash sounds like syphilis. Did you know that the specialty of Dermatology used to be called "Dermatology and Syphilology" because, before antibiotics were invented, the skin doctor was often the first one to diagnose a patient as having syphilis?"

No, Maryellen did not know that, but she did now! A simple blood test confirmed that Dr. Stuart was right.

Another eye-opener occurred when she worked in the Free Clinic. A large number of patients were giving the same name, something simple like "John Doe"—a name commonly being used on charts in many hospitals at that time when the patient had amnesia and the person's identity was unknown. Many of these patients wore expensive clothes and wristwatches and didn't look like they needed a "free" clinic at all.

One such well-dressed man complained of painful urination and pus dripping from the tip of his penis. He winced as Maryellen put a small brush into his urethra to take a sample for laboratory testing.

"Some of these patients have private insurance or could afford to pay full price for an office visit," observed Maryellen's clinic supervisor after the man had left. "But they're ashamed because they would have to admit that they were having sex with someone other than their spouse. They don't want their own doctor to know, so they show up here."

Many of these patients did test positive for a sexually transmitted disease.

Behavior that leads to acquiring certain sexually transmitted diseases (STD) can also lead to serious heart problems. A few generations ago, in the pre-antibiotic era, gonorrhea and syphilis were often associated with serious, life-threatening cardiovascular problems. Both of these STDs can cause inflammation of the heart muscle (myocarditis), which can lead to heart failure. Gonorrhea can also cause infective endocarditis. In its late stages, usually about 10 to 25 years after infection, syphilis can cause an aneurysm of the aorta, predominantly in its first (ascending) part. These "luetic" ascending aortic aneurysms can grow to a massive size, eroding into the breastbone and other nearby bones. They can rupture and cause sudden death. The aneurysm can also extend back to the aortic valve, causing it to leak severely. It can even narrow the openings of the coronary arteries, producing chest pain, a heart attack, or death.

Fortunately, with widespread testing and treatment now available for syphilis and gonorrhea, these complications are now very uncommon. However, another serious STD that causes cardiovascular and other life-threatening problems has arisen in the past few decades. Human immunodeficiency virus (HIV)—the virus that causes AIDS—can damage the heart and its valves in many different ways. HIV infection can lead to an enlarged and weakened heart called a "dilated cardiomyopathy" and heart failure. These problems are at least partly due to myocarditis. HIV infection can also cause isolated abnormal function of the right ventricle, increased pressures within the lungs (pulmonary hypertension), and fluid around the heart—a pericardial effusion.

HIV infection has been associated with premature development of CAD and stroke. It can damage heart valves indirectly by making them more susceptible to endocarditis caused by bacteria and other organisms or by formation of abnormal tissue and blood clots on the valves. HIV infection increases the risk of the heart itself being involved with cancer. These cancers include Kaposi sarcoma and lymphoma, which occur commonly in AIDS patients. Usually the cancer has spread from another part of the body, but it may start in the heart itself. HIV infection can also cause problems with how well the body regulates blood pressure. When a person stands up, blood pressure may fall too much, causing the individual to feel lightheaded or even pass out.

Because one or more of these cardiac problems are commonly seen in people with symptoms related to HIV infection, it has been recommended that they get an echocardiogram at the time of diagnosis to assess for decreased heart function, pericardial effusion, valve disease, or other problems. The echocardiogram can be repeated as needed or at least every one to two years to reevaluate the person.

The most reliable way for a sexually active adult to avoid acquiring these or any kind of sexually transmitted disease is to have a mutually exclusive, monogamous relationship with a sexual partner who also doesn't have any of these diseases. In other situations, condoms certainly provide an increased level of protection, but condoms are not 100% reliable.

When Maryellen started her training as a radiologist over 25 years ago, she and her colleagues were beginning to see unusual cancers and infections in some patients, particularly intravenous drug users and people involved in high-risk sexual behavior. It took the medical community awhile to recognize that a new disease, AIDS, was responsible for these illnesses. The potential for another new, as yet unrecognized sexually transmitted disease to occur in the future will always be with us.

In summary, there are many things you can do and avoid to improve both your cardiac health and your overall health. They do take some effort—but isn't living a longer, healthier, more sexually active life worth it?

Chapter 15 Summary
- ♥ Maintaining a good diet and weight can reduce a person's risk of death and developing heart disease.

- ♥ Regular exercise can reduce the risk of heart problems and improve quality of life, including sex.

- ♥ Small amounts of alcohol may provide mild benefit to the heart. Large amounts of alcohol and any type of tobacco use are harmful to a person's overall health and sex life.

- ♥ Illegal drugs, particularly cocaine, can cause a wide variety of serious and potentially fatal heart problems.

- ♥ Acquired immune deficiency syndrome (AIDS) can cause many types of heart problems, including heart failure and cancers involving the heart.

Chapter 16: Spirituality, Psychology, and Sex
Suggestions for Self-Help

Chapter Preview:
The Power of Prayer
    Physiologic effects of prayer and meditation
    Psychological effects of prayer and meditation
    Effect of prayer on divorce rate
The Effect of Marriage on Heart Health
    Effect on men
    Effect on women
    Negative effect of divorce
    Nourishing your marriage
Coping and Counseling
    Psychologists, counselors, and coaches
Volunteer!
    "Helper's High"
    Positive effect of volunteering
Laughter and Loving
    Physiologic effects of laughter
    Psychological effects of laughter
    Importance of laughter in marriage
Get a Hobby
    Hobbies and your heart
Age Doesn't Matter
    Attitude!

"MAY YOUR HORN be uplifted!" is a quotation from the book of Psalms in the Old Testament.

While it is possible that the "horn" refers to a musical instrument, a more likely interpretation is that it represents the penis! Haven't you heard the term "horny?" Even back in Biblical times, the penis was considered a symbol of strength and health.

Speaking of health . . .

The Power of Prayer

Can prayer help your health—and your heart?

Many physicians and patients are convinced that it can.

For example, prayer and/or meditation can help people handle stress better, which in turn decreases adrenaline (epinephrine) output, leading to decreased blood pressure and heart rate. Because faith in a Supreme Being often gives meaning to life, prayer may also decrease depression, another factor strongly associated with heart disease. A spiritual outlook may also help to decrease hostility and anger. In their teachings, many religions suggest replacing "getting even" with "turning the other cheek" and acting toward others in a positive, less self-destructive way.

For those who attend prayer groups, Bible studies, or church services, there is also the benefit of social interaction, which has been shown to correlate positively with better health outcomes.

Newer neuro-imaging tests have also suggested changes in areas of brain activation when a subject is praying or meditating.

In addition, there are numerous widespread anecdotal reports throughout history of healing or speedy recovery in response to prayer. You or someone you know may have experienced this yourself. The following example is from our own family.

Maryellen's mother needed emergency surgery for a tear (perforation) in her colon that was due to rip-roaring diverticulitis, a type of bowel inflammation. Because her mother has a severe cardiomyopathy (weakness of her heart muscle), the surgeon thought she only had a slim chance of surviving an operation. This would involve doing a colostomy, which means cutting out a piece of bowel and attaching the rest of it to a bag on her side. Without surgery she would most likely die of infection. With a heavy heart, Maryellen and her sister gave the go-ahead for the operation. Maryellen then activated the emergency telephone prayer chain at our church.

Within an hour, over two hundred people were praying for Maryellen's mother. They also prayed for guidance and wisdom for her surgeon and the other members of the medical team. Our prayer chain routinely prays for the doctors, nurses, and other healthcare providers caring for the patient, because we believe God uses them as His instruments.

After the procedure was completed, one of the nurses remarked how amazing it was that Mom sailed right through the operation. The surgeon had been able to immediately locate the tear in the colon—something that can be extremely difficult to do with all of the inflammation there. Then he was able to quickly repair it without having to put in the colostomy that had been planned. Mom is still alive today.

On the other hand, it is sometimes difficult to confirm the power of prayer by means of scientific studies. For example, a recent study concerning prayer was reported by Dr. Herbert Benson and colleagues in the April 2006 issue of the *American Heart Journal*. Dr. Benson, author of *The Relaxation Response*, is a highly-respected cardiologist and Co-Director of the Mind/Body Medical Institute affiliated with Harvard Medical School. The article was entitled, "Study of the Therapeutic Effects of Intercessory Prayer (STEP) in Cardiac Bypass Patients: A Multicenter Randomized

Trial of Uncertainty and Certainty of Receiving Intercessory Prayer." (Whew! That was a mouthful!)

In this study, having intercessors pray for patients had no effect on their recovery from coronary artery bypass surgery. In fact, if patients knew the intercessor group was praying for them, they actually had a higher rate of complications than patients who didn't know for sure whether they were being prayed for!

Why the above results occurred is uncertain. As the authors rightly point out, it is quite possible—even extremely likely—that all of the patients, including the control group, were praying for themselves and had family and personal friends praying for them as well. It would have been unethical as well as impossible to prevent that from occurring. Since not all of the variable factors could be controlled, this may have affected the outcome of the study.

Doctors who recommend prayer in the medical setting need to be sure that the patient does not equate illness or lack of recovery with punishment from God.

Whether or not you believe that prayer can help physical improvement in an illness, one thing is pretty much agreed upon: prayer usually does help the patient and his or her family cope. Here's another example based on our own experience.

One day a mammography technologist told Maryellen that a female patient had a special request. This woman had recently been diagnosed as having an abnormal area in one of her breasts that could be a cancer. Maryellen was going to do a "needle localization" procedure on her. Before the advent of newer "stereotactic" techniques, all of these procedures were done with a woman sitting down and required a considerable amount of cooperation from the woman herself. Using the patient's mammogram to guide her,

Maryellen would insert a thin needle into the woman's breast until the tip of the needle was at the abnormal area. A surgeon would then cut out ("biopsy") a sample of breast tissue containing the abnormal area, guided by where the tip of the needle showed this abnormality was located.

Before having this stressful needle localization, the anxious woman asked if Maryellen would pray with her. Maryellen was happy to do this. After their prayer was finished, the woman became noticeably more relaxed. The procedure went smoothly.

In the days that followed this incident, many of the other technologists also began asking Maryellen to pray with patients. She was puzzled why all of these requests started flowing in suddenly.

"Many people tell us they believe that prayer can help them," explained one astute technologist. "Haven't you noticed how the patients act less stressed after you pray with them? Hardly anyone faints any more, we use less local anesthetic to numb the skin, and the procedures go faster and smoother."

In addition to its effect on health and well-being, prayer also helps to divorce-proof a couple. The national divorce rate hovers around 50%. Statistics given by Robert A. Ruhnke in his book *For Better and For Ever* show that if a couple attends church services together once a week, the divorce rate drops to as low as 3%. If they pray together in their home regularly, the divorce rate plummets to as low as 0.3%.

That brings us to the next question: Is a healthy marriage good for your heart, and why?

The Effect of Marriage on Heart Health

Marriage plays an important role in physical as well as psychological health, especially for men.

"There's plenty of evidence that human sexuality, intimacy, love, and marriage are very, very good for our health," says Dr. Stephen Bogdewic, Executive Associate Dean and Professor of Family Medicine at Indiana University School of Medicine.

Here are some examples that support Dr. Bogdewic's statement. In general, married men live healthier and longer lives compared to single men. (And no, it's not just that their lives seem longer!)

A man's wife and family form a social support system for him, which in turn helps keep stress hormones low. Also, a wife may see that her husband eats better than an unmarried man. (Well, there are always exceptions—Henry knows Maryellen isn't much of a cook!) Married men may engage in less risky behaviors such as getting drunk or skydiving. In addition, the wives of married men may see to it that their spouses take their medications regularly and follow their doctor's advice.

Women also derive health benefits from marriage. However, research studies indicate they are more likely to achieve those benefits if the marriage is a good one compared to a bad one. A study in the *Journal of the American Medical Association* published in December 2000 evaluated women who had experienced a heart attack or unstable angina. Women who had a stressful relationship with a male partner were nearly three times more likely to have another heart attack or other cardiac event than those whose relationship was not stressful. Divorce has also been reported to have worse health effects on women than on men.

Another study published in the *American Journal of Cardiology* in 2001 assessed the effects of marital stress on men and women with congestive heart failure. Those individuals who were happily married lived longer than those in unhappy marriages.

Both heart rate and blood pressure can rise during arguments, triggered by stress. Therefore, for physical as well as psychological reasons, a couple might consider counseling in order to improve their marital situation as well as their heart health.

Jennifer Baker, Psy.D., is director of the Marriage and Family Therapy Program at Forest Institute of Professional Psychology in Springfield, Misssouri. She has a wealth of clinical experience in this area and oversees the training of providers of mental health services. We interviewed her about marriage and divorce issues.

"Some people think the way to avoid the negative effects of a difficult marriage relationship is to find someone else. In fact, many times, people are much better off working on the relationship that they have," says Dr. Baker. "Please know that I certainly would not endorse someone staying in a marriage where one is being beaten, abused, or where one's partner is habitually unfaithful. I'm simply lamenting the ease with which people get out of marriages that might have succeeded had they gotten help and worked at it. There is ample evidence that divorce negatively impacts both men and women's lives, even if they are happily remarried."

We also asked Dr. Baker about couples who live together instead of marrying in order to avoid the problems that accompany going through a divorce.

"Living together instead of marrying does not eliminate psychological problems that arise when a couple breaks up," says Dr. Baker. "In fact, I sometimes refer to this as a 'pre-marital divorce.'"

Nourish your marriage. Make it a priority in your life. Show your spouse that your relationship is important to you. Study and read about healthy marriages. Attend a talk on relationships or even a marriage course. These might be offered at a church, a school or college, or another local or out-of-town location. Even the best marriage benefits from continuing education. When we lived in St. Louis, we regularly attended Marriage Encounter meetings and Marriage Encounter weekends to enhance our communication as a couple.

Here in our new home in southwest Missouri, Maryellen volunteers for a wonderful nonprofit organization called Ozarks Marriage Matters (OMM). OMM educates and promotes healthy marriages in our community and the surrounding area. It has a regular newsletter with helpful information that can be accessed on its website, which you can find when you visit: www.ozarksmarriagematters.org. Very useful information on healthy marriages can also be found at www.smartmarriages.com. The Administration for Children and Families is also a good resource. Its website is www.acf.hhs.gov.

Janice Kielcolt-Glaser, Ph.D., Professor of Psychiatry and Psychology at Ohio State University College of Medicine, has done research showing that wounds heal faster in couples involved in happy rather than hostile relationships. This suggests that it may benefit you to work on your marriage as part of an overall cardiac rehabilitation program following a heart attack or heart surgery.

As with other serious illnesses, there is often a "hidden patient" when heart disease is present. This refers to a spouse or sometimes another family member or caregiver who develops depression, anxiety, or other psychological or even physical sickness because of his or her mate's illness. Asking how this other person is "holding up" and providing for his or her needs is also important.

Joining a support group may also help you as a married couple and as a heart patient. Support groups and supportive people decrease your stress level and improve your coping skills. The social interaction a support group provides may also help depression.

Coping and Counseling
Behavioral medicine programs and mental health professionals such as psychologists, social workers, and counselors may help patients identify and reduce sources of stress in their lives. The psychological effects of heart problems, including depression and anxiety, can sometimes be more devastating than the physical effects. Changing stress-producing behaviors and maintaining positive thinking patterns can improve quality of life for both the patient and the patient's partner.

There is a new movement called Positive Psychology that focuses on what individuals do well and on what they can do to improve or enhance their lives. Sometimes people who are reluctant to undergo traditional psychotherapy may be open to speaking with a "life coach" who can help them greatly improve their situation.

Volunteer!
Have you ever heard of "helper's high?" It is another effect that researchers feel may be due to oxytocin (remember chapter 3?).

"Volunteering is good for your heart and your health," says Stephen G. Post, Ph.D., professor of Bioethics at Maryellen's alma mater, Case Western

Reserve University School of Medicine in Cleveland, Ohio.

"People who 'do for others' generally live healthier and longer lives."

Dr. Post has extensively studied the practice of altruism. Altruism means showing compassion, kindness, or generosity toward other people. Over 20 peer-reviewed medical studies support his opinion. His only caveat or caution is to patients or caregivers who may already feel overburdened or overworked. In that case, they might find volunteering too stressful. However, if their condition or situation permits, volunteering will frequently help them as well as the person who is being helped.

For those who wish to learn more about this fascinating topic, it is discussed further in the book *It's Good to Be Good* by Stephen G. Post, Ph.D., with Jill Niemark, May 2007, Random House.

Volunteering is also an activity that can be done either as an individual or as a couple. Working together for a good cause can enhance your relationship with each other.

Laughter and Loving

Laughter helps to defuse tension both in and out of the bedroom. Although it may cause some increase in heart rate, it can decrease blood pressure, stress hormones, and muscle tension.

Michael Miller, M.D., Director of Preventive Cardiology at the University of Maryland, presented his research on laughter at the American College of Cardiology meeting in March 2005. Ultrasound was used to study the size of certain blood vessels. After watching a funny movie, 19 out of 20 volunteers showed good effects on their blood vessels, with the average artery diameter increasing 22% during laughter. After watching a stressful movie, blood flow worsened in 14 out of 20, with the average artery diameter decreasing 35%.

Dr. Lee Berk and other researchers have done studies suggesting that laughter may increase the number of germ-killing cells in the body and improve the immune system. Laughter may also help to prevent inflammation of the endothelium (inner lining) of blood vessels, potentially decreasing the risk of developing coronary artery disease.

Laughter also decreases depression and may replace feelings of irritability and anger with healthier emotions.

Just as a married couple may schedule time for sex, they should schedule time for laughter. Both activities decrease stress and help solidify the relationship.

Maryellen attended a psychology course recently at nearby Missouri State University, taught by the noted Russian comedian Yakov Smirnoff. Yakov has a popular theater in nearby Branson, Missouri, a favorite destination in the Ozarks for travelers.

Yakov has a master's degree in Positive Psychology from the University of Pennsylvania. He gave his students, ranging from eighteen to over eighty years of age, many insights into love and relationships in his course, "Happily Ever Laughter." He shared the view that laughter is a gauge or barometer of the state of a couple's marriage. When a couple stops laughing together, it suggests that the relationship is in trouble. This loss of laughter may even occur before problems with sex arise.

Laughter and opportunities for laughter are good for relationships and for the heart. Sharing jokes, watching humorous television shows together, or reading funny articles and books may also be helpful. You may enjoy the book *How to Commit Monogamy: A Lighthearted Look at Long-Term Love*, by Elaine Viets, one of Maryellen's favorite authors. Elaine's articles and books always evoke smiles.

Get a Hobby
Making time for a hobby or a favorite pastime may help your heart by relieving stress. It may also give you something interesting to discuss with your partner. If you don't have a partner, it may help you meet someone with similar interests.

Hobbies range from fishing to photography, stamp collecting to sports. Listening to music, playing a musical instrument, and engaging in artistic endeavors such as painting or sculpting are also great hobbies. Almost everybody can find an activity that suits him or her. Check for ideas at a library or community college. We do, however, recommend being cautious about emotionally or physically strenuous hobbies such as bungee jumping. Common sense is the key.

Henry's hobbies include model rocketry, electronics, astronomy, and writing science fiction. Maryellen's hobbies involve shopping at the mall and attending writers' group meetings. She also loves watching television programs or reading magazines that feature stories on people. It's a welcome break from her usual medical journals.

Age Doesn't Matter
An 88-year-old man went to the doctor's office for a check-up. The man asked the doctor if he could have a sperm count done.

Knowing that people can have sex well into old age, the doctor handed him a small jar. He told him to bring back the "specimen" when he returned at his next visit.

When the octogenarian returned the following week, he handed the doctor the container. It was empty.

The doctor looked at him quizzically.

"Well, Doc," said the patient. "This is what happened. First I tried with my right hand. Then I tried with my left hand. Then my wife tried with her right hand. Then she tried with her left hand. And neither of us could get the lid off that jar!"

Here's to living, laughing, and loving for many years to come!

Chapter 16 Summary

- ♥ Prayer may have positive effects on health and well-being, particularly by improving one's ability to cope with stress. It also has a positive effect on marriage and relationships.

- ♥ In general, married men live healthier and longer lives compared to single men.

- ♥ Women also derive health benefits from marriage, but they are more likely to achieve those benefits in a good marriage rather than a bad one.

- ♥ Behavioral medicine programs and mental health professionals such as psychologists, counselors, and coaches may improve quality of life for patients and their partners.

♥ Engaging in volunteer work, laughter, and hobbies may also improve heart health and relationships.

Table 1. Common Symptoms and Treatments of Major Cardiovascular Diseases

Disease	Symptoms	Treatment
Coronary artery disease	Chest pain or pressure (discomfort may go into the neck or left arm) Shortness of breath Fatigue	Beta-blockers Calcium antagonists Nitrates Ranolazine Aspirin Clopidogrel ACE inhibitors and ARBs if heart function is moderately to severely decreased Coronary angioplasty Coronary artery bypass graft surgery Transmyocardial laser revascularization External enhanced counterpulsation
Heart failure	Shortness of breath—may occur with or without activity; may cause a person to wake up at night Fatigue and weakness Fluid retention with swelling of the ankles (edema) or belly (ascites)	ACE inhibitors ARBs Beta-blockers Diuretics Digoxin Nitrates Hydralazine
Heart valve disease		

Aortic regurgitation	Shortness of breath
	Chest pain
	Fatigue
	Palpitations
		Calcium antagonists:
		  Nifedipine
		  Felodipine
		  Amlodipine
		ACE inhibitors
		ARBs
		Hydralazine
		Valve replacement in severe cases

Table 1

Condition	Symptoms	Treatment
Aortic stenosis	Chest pain Shortness of breath Syncope (passing out)	Aortic valve replacement if aortic stenosis is severe and reduced heart function or symptoms are present

Mitral regurgitation	Shortness of breath
	Fatigue and weakness
		Calcium antagonists
		  Nifedipine
		  Felodipine
		  Amlodipine
		ACE inhibitors
		ARBs
		Hydralazine
		Valve replacement or repair in severe cases

Mitral stenosis	Shortness of breath
	Chest pain
	Palpitations
	Coughing up blood
	Hoarseness
	Transient ischemic attack or stroke
		Diuretics
		To treat rapid heart rate:
		  Beta-blockers
		  Diltiazem
		  Verapamil
		  Digoxin (if atrial fibrillation or flutter is present)
		Warfarin (if evidence of blood clots or if atrial fibrillation or flutter is present)
		Valve replacement or valvotomy in severe cases

High Blood Pressure (Hypertension)	Usually no symptoms except those due to problems caused by hypertension, such as coronary artery disease, stroke, or damage to the kidneys	Beta-blockers
		Calcium antagonists
		ACE inhibitors
		ARBs
		Diuretics
		Miscellaneous agents:
		  Methyldopa
		  Clonidine
		  Prazosin
		  Doxazosin
		  Terazosin
		  Minoxidil
		  Hydralazine
		Reduce salt intake
		Exercise

Table 1

Arrhythmias

Bradyarrhythmias (abnormally slow heart rate)	Fatigue Shortness of breath Lightheadedness Syncope	Pacemaker

Atrial flutter and fibrillation	Palpitations
	Fatigue
	Shortness of breath
	Lightheadedness
	Syncope
	Stroke
		Medications to reduce heart rate:
		  Beta-blockers
		  Calcium antagonists
		    Diltiazem
		    Verapamil
		  Digoxin
		Warfarin
		Aspirin
		Antiarrhythmic agents
		  Flecainide
		  Propafenone
		  Sotalol
		  Amiodarone
		Ablation procedures
		Maze procedure
		Cardioversion (electrical shock to the heart)

PACs and PVCs	Palpitations Chest discomfort Lightheadedness	Avoid or reduce use of alcohol and caffeine Avoid medications that stimulate the heart, such as pseudoephedrine (Sudafed) Low dose of beta-blocker, diltiazem, or verapamil

PSVT	Palpitations
	Shortness of breath
	Chest pain
	Lightheadedness
	Syncope
		"Straining" maneuvers
		Adenosine
		Beta-blocker
		Calcium antagonists:
		  Diltiazem
		  Verapamil
		Cardioversion

Table 1

Ventricular tachycardia	Depending on heart rate and how long the arrhythmia lasts, may produce:
	No symptoms
	Chest pain
	Shortness of breath
	Palpitations,
	Lightheadedness
	Syncope
	Death
		Medications:
		  Lidocaine
		  Amiodarone
		  Procainamide
		Cardioversion
		Implantable cardioverter-defibrillator for long-term prevention

Carotid artery or other cerebrovascular disease	Signs and symptoms of a TIA or stroke, such as: Sudden weakness or numbness in an arm or leg Loss of vision Difficulty speaking	Aspirin Clopidogrel Warfarin Thrombolytic therapy (within 3 hours of onset of stroke symptoms) Carotid endarterectomy Carotid angioplasty and stent placement
Peripheral arterial disease	Blockages in the arteries of the legs can cause: Pain in the calves or buttocks Reddish or bluish discoloration of the feet Numbness or weakness of the legs Cold feet or legs Hair loss on the feet and legs	Aspirin Clopidogrel Warfarin Cilostazol Pentoxifylline Cholesterol-lowering medications Calcium antagonists Angioplasty and stent placement Bypass surgery

ACE inhibitor = angiotensin-converting enzyme inhibitor;
ARB = angiotensin receptor blocker;
PAC = premature atrial contraction;
PVC = premature ventricular contraction;
PSVT = paroxysmal supraventricular tachycardia;
TIA = transient ischemic attack.

Table 2. Major Types of Cardiovascular Medicines

Class	Primary uses	Examples (Trade name in parentheses)
Beta-blockers	AF, CAD, HBP, HF, MI	Propranolol (Inderal) Metoprolol (Lopressor, Toprol XL) Atenolol (Tenormin) Carvedilol (Coreg)
Calcium antagonists	CAD, HBP AF—verapamil and diltiazem only	Verapamil (Calan, Isoptin, Covera-HS) Diltiazem (Cardizem, Dilacor XR, Tiazac, Cartia XT) Nifedipine (Adalat CC, Procardia XL) Felodipine (Plendil) Amlodipine (Norvasc)
Nitrates	CAD, HF	Nitroglycerin (Nitrostat, Nitro-Bid) Isosorbide mononitrate (Imdur) Isosorbide dinitrate (Isordil)
Angiotensin-converting enzyme Inhibitors (ACE inhibitors)	CAD, HBP, HF, MI	Captopril (Capoten) Lisinopril (Prinvil, Zestril) Enalapril (Vasotec) Quinapril (Accupril) Ramipril (Altace) Fosinopril (Monopril) Trandolapril (Mavik, Tarka) Benazepril (Lotensin)
Angiotensin receptor blockers (ARBs)	CAD, HBP, HF	Losartan (Cozaar) Valsartan (Diovan) Irbesartan (Avapro) Candesartan (Atacand) Olmesartan (Benicar)
Digitalis	AF, HF	Digoxin (Lanoxin, Digitek)

Table 2

Hypolipidemic agents	Elevated cholesterol		HMG-CoA reductase inhibitors
			  Lovastatin (Mevacor, Altoprev)
			  Pravastatin (Pravachol)
			  Simvastatin (Zocor)
			  Atorvastatin (Lipitor)
			  Rosuvastatin (Crestor)
			
			Bile acid sequestrants:
			  Cholestyramine (Questran)
			  Colestipol (Colestid)
			  Colesevelam (WelChol)
			
			Fibrates:
			  Gemfibrozil (Lopid)
			  Fenofibrate (Tricor)
			
			Others:
			  Niacin (Niaspan)
			  Ezetimibe (Zetia)
			  Simvastatin + ezetimibe (Vytorin)

Antiarrhythmics	AF, PSVT, VT		Quinidine (Quinaglute)
			Procainamide (Pronestyl, Procan SR)
			Flecainide (Tambocor)
			Propafenone (Rythmol)
			Amiodarone (Pacerone, Cordarone)
			Sotalol (Betapace)
			VT only:
			  Lidocaine (Xylocaine)
			  Mexilitene (Mexitil)
			  Tocainide (Tonocard)

Diuretics	HBP, HF		Hydrochlorothiazide Metolazone (Zaroxolyn) Furosemide (Lasix) Bumetanide (Bumex) Torsemide (Demadex) Spironolactone (Aldactone) Amiloride

Table 2

Antiplatelet agents	AF, CAD, MI	Aspirin Clopidogrel (Plavix) Ticlopidine (Ticlid)
Anticoagulants	AF, CAD, HF, MI	Warfarin (Coumadin) Heparin Enoxaparin (Lovenox) Dalteparin (Fragmin)
Thrombolytics	Acute MI	Streptokinase (Streptase) Alteplase (Activase) Reteplase (Retavase) Tenecteplase (TNKase)
Other	CAD	Ranolazine (Ranexa)

AF = atrial fibrillation and atrial flutter;
CAD = coronary artery disease;
HBP = high blood pressure;
HF = heart failure;
MI = myocardial infarction;
PSVT = paroxysmal supraventricular tachycardia;
VT = ventricular tachycardia.

Glossary and Definitions of Acronyms

Angina pectoris: Chest pain due to an area of the heart not getting enough blood.

Aorta: The major artery that comes off the heart. The aorta sends blood rich in oxygen to the rest of the body.

Aortic valve: The heart valve that regulates the flow of the blood out from the left ventricle into the aorta.

Atherosclerosis: Blockages in arteries due to injury to their inner lining. Atherosclerosis can be caused by high blood pressure, smoking, diabetes, and elevated blood cholesterol.

Atrial fibrillation: An abnormal heart rhythm beginning in an atrium that generates many hundreds of impulses per minute. Atrial fibrillation usually causes an abnormally fast and irregular heartbeat.

Atrial flutter: An abnormal heart rhythm beginning in an atrium that produces up to about 250 to 350 beats per minute. Atrial flutter usually causes an abnormally fast heartbeat.

Bradyarrhythmia: An abnormally slow (less than 60 beats/minute) heart rhythm.

Cerebrovascular accident: (See Stroke).

Cervix: The neck or "spout" of the uterus, located in uppermost, deepest part of the vagina. The cervix allows fluids to pass between the uterus and the vagina.

Clitoris: Erectile tissue located just above the urethra and the opening of a woman's vagina. The clitoris provides pleasurable sensations when stimulated.

Coronary angiography: Injection of X-ray contrast ("dye") directly into the arteries of the heart to check for blockages.

Coronary angioplasty: Procedure used to open up a blocked coronary artery by inflating a balloon within the blockage.

Coronary artery: One of the three blood vessels—the right coronary artery and the two branches of the left coronary artery (the left anterior descending artery and circumflex artery)—that supply blood to the heart.

Coronary artery disease (CAD): Blockage in one or more arteries supplying blood to the heart. This blockage is usually due to atherosclerosis.

Coronary artery bypass graft surgery (CABG): Surgery using veins from the legs or arteries (usually from the chest) to "bypass" blocked coronary arteries and supply more blood to the heart.

Coronary artery stent: A small metal mesh used to keep a blocked coronary artery open after coronary angioplasty or a similar procedure.

Echocardiogram: A test for taking pictures of the heart and its valves and evaluating blood flow using ultrasonic waves.

Electrocardiogram (EKG): A test used to record the heart's electrical activity.

Endometrium: The tissue lining the inner wall of the uterus that provides blood and nutrients to a fertilized egg.

Estrogen: The main female sex hormone. Estrogen is needed to make a woman's sex organs mature during puberty and to make egg cells become capable of being fertilized.

Erectile dysfunction (ED): Inability of a man to achieve and sustain an erection long enough to complete sexual intercourse.

Fallopian tubes: The tubes that connect a woman's ovaries to her uterus, allowing a fertilized egg to reach the uterus and grow there into a baby.

Fertilization: The uniting of a woman's ovum (egg cell) and a man's sperm cell to form a baby.

Implantable cardioverter-defibrillator (ICD): A device placed beneath the skin that senses the presence of a serious, abnormally fast heart rhythm and shocks the heart back to regular rhythm.

HDL cholesterol: High-density lipoprotein cholesterol, "good" cholesterol. The risk of developing coronary artery disease and atherosclerosis in other blood vessels increases as levels of HDL cholesterol fall below normal.

Heart failure (HF): Inability of the heart to provide enough blood to meet the body's needs, usually caused by weakness or increased stiffness of the left ventricle.

LDL cholesterol: Low-density lipoprotein cholesterol, "bad" cholesterol. The risk of developing coronary artery disease as well as atherosclerosis in other blood vessels increases as levels of LDL cholesterol rise above normal.

Left atrium (LA): The upper chamber on the left side of the heart. The left atrium directs blood through the mitral valve into the left ventricle.

Left ventricle (LV): The lower chamber on the left side of the heart. The left ventricle is the main pumping chamber of the heart.

Mitral valve: The heart valve that regulates blood flow between the left atrium and the left ventricle. It has two leaflets while the other heart valves have three.

Myocardial infarction (MI): Permanent damage to part of the heart, usually due to severely reduced blood flow caused by coronary artery disease.

Myocardial perfusion imaging (MPI): Use of a mildly radioactive material injected into a vein during a stress test to assess blood flow to the heart and the presence of coronary artery disease.

Myocardial ischemia: Reduction of blood supply below the level heart muscle needs to function properly.

Myocardium: Heart muscle.

Oocyte: An immature egg cell.

Ovaries: The two reproductive organs in a woman's pelvis that produce female hormones as well as egg cells (ova) needed to make a baby.

Ovum: The egg cell that is a woman's contribution to making a baby.

Pacemaker: A device for generating electrical impulses to make a heart chamber contract and produce a heartbeat.

Penis: The external male sex organ. The penis ejaculates sperm cells into a woman's vagina for fertilization of an egg and reproduction.

Placenta: A flat circular organ that develops in the uterus during pregnancy, attaching a developing baby to its mother through the umbilical cord.

Progesterone: One of the female sex hormones.

Pulmonary embolism: A blood clot in an artery of the lung.

Pulmonic valve: The heart valve that regulates blood flow between the right ventricle and the pulmonary artery.

Right atrium (RA): The upper chamber on the right side of the heart. The right atrium receives blood from the veins and directs it through the tricuspid valve into the right ventricle.

Right ventricle (RV): The lower chamber on the right side of the heart. The right ventricle pumps blood to the lungs.

Scrotum: The skin-covered pouch beneath the penis that contains the testes.

Sperm cells (spermatozoa): The cells that are the man's contribution to making a baby.

Stroke (cerebrovascular accident): Damage to a part of the brain caused by not enough blood and oxygen getting to it.

Tachyarrhythmia: An abnormally fast (more than 100 beats/minute) heart rhythm.

Testes: Paired male sex organs, a man's equivalent to a woman's ovaries. The testes produce testosterone and sperm cells.

Testosterone: The main male sex hormone. Testosterone is needed to make a man's sex organs mature during puberty and to produce sperm cells.

Thrombus: A blood clot.

Tricuspid valve: The heart valve that regulates blood flow between the right atrium and the right ventricle.

Umbilical cord: The cord containing blood vessels that connects the mother to the baby during pregnancy.

Uterus (Womb): The pear-shaped organ in a woman's pelvis where a baby grows during pregnancy.

Ventricular assist device (VAD): A mechanical device used to support a weakened heart by helping pump blood.

Vagina: The muscular sheath in a woman's pelvis that allows entry of the penis for sexual intercourse and reproduction.

Ventricular fibrillation (VF): An abnormal fast (often over 400 beats/minute) heart rhythm that makes the ventricles quiver (fibrillate) instead of contracting and pumping blood.

Ventricular tachycardia (VT): An abnormally fast (110 to 400 beats/minute) heart rhythm originating in a ventricle.

References and Suggested Reading

Cardiovascular Medicine:

1. *Braunwald's Heart Disease: A Textbook of Cardiovascular Medicine*, Seventh Edition, edited by Eugene Braunwald et al. W. B. Saunders Company, 2005.

2. *Feigenbaum's Echocardiography*, Sixth Edition, edited by Harvey Feigenbaum, William F. Armstrong, and Thomas Ryan. Lippincott Williams & Wilkins, 2004.

3. *Nuclear Cardiac Imaging: Principles and Applications*, Third Edition, edited by Ami Iskandrian and Mario Verani. Oxford University Press, 2003.

5. *Grossman's Cardiac Catheterization, Angiography, and Intervention*, edited by Donald Baim. Lippincott Williams and Wilkins, 2005.

4. *Cardiac Surgery*, Third Edition, edited by Nicholas Kouchoukos, Eugene Blackstone, Donald Doty, et al. Churchill Livingstone, 2003.

5. Lichtenstein AH, et al. Diet and Lifestyle Recommendations Revision 2006: A Scientific Statement from the American Heart Association Nutrition Committee. Circulation 2006;114:82–96.

6. Thom T, et al. Heart Disease and Stroke Statistics—2006 Update: A Report From the American Heart Association Statistics Committee and Stroke Statistics Subcommittee. Circulation 2006; 113:e85–e151.

7. DeBusk R, Drory Y, Goldstein I, et al. Management of sexual dysfunction in patients with cardiovascular disease: recommendations of the Princeton Consensus Panel. American Journal of Cardiology 2000;86: 175–81.

8. *Hurst's The Heart*, Eleventh Edition, edited by Valentin Fuster, R. Wayne Alexander, and Robert A. O'Rourke. McGraw-Hill, 2004.

9. *Physicians' Desk Reference*, Sixtieth Edition. Thomson PDR, 2006.

Reproductive Medicine:

1. *Novak's Gynecology*, Thirteenth Edition. Jonathan S. Berek, editor. Lippincott Williams and Wilkins, 2002.

2. *Campbell's Urology*, Eighth Edition, edited by Patrick C. Walsh, Alan B. Retik, E. Darracott Vaughn, et al. Saunders, 2002.

3. *Williams Textbook of Endocrinology*, Tenth Edition, edited by P. Reed Larsen, Henry M. Kronenberg, Schlomo Melded, et al. Saunders, 2002.

4. *Kaplan and Sadock's Comprehensive Textbook of Psychiatry*, Eighth Edition, edited by Benjamin J. Sadock and Virginia A. Sadock. Lippincott Williams and Wilkins, 2004.

5. Grady D. Management of menopausal symptoms. New England Journal of Medicine 2006;355:2338-47.

Psychology, Marriage, and Spirituality

1. *The Case for Marriage: Why Married People are Happier, Healthier, and Better Off Financially* by Linda J. Waite and Maggie Gallagher. Doubleday, 2000.

2. *Receiving Love: Transform Your Relationship by Letting Yourself Be Loved* by Harville Hendrix and Helen LaKelly Hunt. Atria Books, 2004.

3. *The Truth About Love: The Highs, the Lows, and How You Can Make It Last Forever* by Dr. Patricia Love. Fireside, 2001.

4. *Rekindling Desire: A Step-by-Step Program to Help Low-Sex and No-Sex Marriages* by Barry McCarthy and Emily McCarthy. Brunner-Routledge, 2003.

5. *Love is a Decision* by Gary Smalley and John Trent. W Publishing Group, 2001.

6. *Lasting Love: The 5 Secrets of Growing a Vital, Conscious Relationship* by Gay Hendricks and Kathlyn Hendricks. Rodale, 2004.

7. *Ten Lessons to Transform Your Marriage* by John Gottman, Julie Schwartz-Gottman, and Joan Declaire. Crown Publishers, 2006.

8. *Fighting for Your Marriage* by Howard J. Markman, Scott M. Stanley, and Susan L. Blumberg. John Wiley and Sons, Inc., 2001.

Index

Abciximab, 193
Ablation, 218
Accelerated idioventricular rhythm, 107
Accelerated junctional rhythm, 107
Acquired immune deficiency syndrome (AIDS), 55, 314, 319–321
Adrenaline, 57, 293, 324
Alcohol, 79, 107, 233, 309, 313, 315, 321
Alpha-blocker(s), 242, 249
Alprostadil, 243
Alteplase, 133
Altruism, 332
American Heart Association (AHA), 298–300, 303
Amiloride, 175, 176, 273
Amiodarone, 126, 127, 177, 242, 274, 278
Amlodipine, 175, 236
Amyl nitrate, 116
Andropause, 41
Anemia, 41, 82, 155, 164, 273
Aneurysm
  aortic
    abdominal, 89, 90, 93, 171, 172, 207
    ascending, 91, 92, 318
    thoracic, 90, 91
  left ventricular, 153, 154
  luetic (syphilitic), 318
  of arteries in the brain, 264
Angina pectoris, 73–77, 96, 97, 119, 127, 130, 140, 173, 177, 195, 221, 234, 235, 239, 248–250, 288, 290, 328
Angiography, coronary, 132–139, 169, 170, 172,

189, 191, 208, 261, 279, 292, 293, 346
sex and, 222
Angioplasty
   coronary, 83, 129, 135, 136, 140, 188, 189, 193, 195, 198, 200, 217, 219, 222, 227, 248, 294, 346
      restenosis after, 192, 193
      sex and, 222, 227, 248, 249
      women and, 260, 261, 290
   other arteries, 172
Angioscopy, 192
Angiotensin receptor blockers (ARBs), 122, 155, 157, 173, 238, 274
Angiotensin-converting enzyme (ACE) inhibitors, 121, 122, 154, 155, 173, 175, 180, 238, 242, 274, 275, 292
Ankle-brachial index, 172
Antiarrhythmics, 126, 178
Antibiotics, 98, 101, 102, 184, 194, 317
Anticoagulants. *See* Blood thinners.
Antihistamines, 233
Antihypertensives. *See* Blood pressure medications.
Anxiety, 57, 84, 226, 232, 257, 304, 330, 331
Aorta, 345
   anatomy of, 63, 64, 67, 86
   aneurysm of. *See* Aneurysm, aortic.
   blood clots and, 88
   blood pressure and, 66
   dissection of. *See* Dissection, aortic.
Aortic regurgitation, 97–100, 175, 237, 238, 270, 271
Aortic stenosis, 80, 96, 100, 135, 204, 206, 207, 270
Aortic valve, 345
   bicuspid, 96, 262, 263
   function of, 62

Appendage, left atrial, 143, 144, 206
Arteriogram, 172, 246
Artery (ies)
  carotid, 86–88, 93, 168, 171, 174, 208
  femoral, 134, 200
  internal mammary, 197, 198
Artificial heart. *See* Heart, artificial.
Artificial heart valves. *See* Valves, artificial.
Asexual reproduction, 52, 53
Aspirin, 87, 93, 119–121, 133, 154, 157, 172, 174, 183, 193, 239, 274, 278
Asystole, 106
Atenolol, 121, 234, 274
Atherectomy, 190–192, 219
Atherosclerosis, 72, 93, 184, 245, 296, 298, 301, 345, 346, 347, 348
Atorvastatin, 182, 275
Atrial fibrillation, 99, 100, 108–111, 127, 162–164, 173–178, 218, 236, 239, 269, 270, 291
Atrial flutter, 108, 110, 164, 174, 177, 178, 218, 236, 239
Atrial myxoma. *See* Myxoma.
Atrial septal defect, 104, 209, 262, 266
Atrioventricular (AV) node, 66, 105–111
Atrium (atria), 62–66, 88, 104, 105–111, 125, 161–163, 178, 218, 256, 345, 348, 350
Auscultation, 161
Automatic external defibrillator (AED), 123
Baker, Dr. Jennifer, 329
Barnard, Dr. Christian, 210
Behavioral medicine, 331, 335
Benazepril, 122, 274
Benson, Dr. Herbert, 325
Berk, Dr. Lee, 333
Beta-blocker(s), 107, 121, 150, 154, 157, 170, 175,

177–179, 234–238, 242, 251, 270, 273, 274, 286, 294
Biopsy
  breast, 327
  endomyocardial, 210
Birth control, 114, 287, 294
  pills, 85, 113, 285, 310
  types, 45
Bisoprolol, 274
Bivalirudin, 193
Blood pressure
  AIDS and, 319
  amphetamines and, 314
  aortic dissection and, 90, 91
  cocaine and, 312, 313
  definition of, 66
  diastolic, 66, 84, 255
  exercise and, 66, 67, 305
  laughter and, 332
  low, 82, 127, 131, 132, 153, 161, 166, 179, 213, 225, 242, 256
  medications and, 119, 121, 122, 173–179, 236, 241, 242, 308
  oxytocin and, 57
  prayer and, 324
  pregnancy and, 255–260, 263, 270, 271
  pulmonary embolism and, 114
  sex and, 221, 246, 247, 250
  stress test and, 140, 141, 149, 150, 156, 329
  systolic, 66, 84, 172
Blood pressure medications. *See also* Tables 1 and 2, 85, 242, 259
Blood thinners, 120, 154, 155, 174, 193, 239, 244, 271, 272, 275
Body mass index, 302, 303

Bogdewic, Dr. Stephen, 328
Brachytherapy, 195
Bradyarrhythmia, 105
Bradycardia, 105
Breastfeeding
 and cardiac medications, 277, 278
 and oxytocin, 57
Bruit, 161
Bumetanide, 176, 238
Caffeine, 107, 150
Calcium, 72, 93, 169, 175, 177, 189, 206, 249, 273, 275, 276, 301
Calcium antagonist. See Calcium channel blockers.
Calcium channel blockers, 183, 236, 286
Calorie(s), 155, 288, 298, 300, 303, 304
Cancer, 32, 55, 102–104, 113, 114, 211, 246, 261, 279, 283, 284, 309, 310, 319, 326
Candesartan, 122, 274
Captopril, 122, 274
Carbohydrates, 300
Carbon dioxide, 63, 64, 113
Cardiac catheterization, 25, 135, 293
Cardiomyopathy, 258
 dilated, 319
 hypertrophic obstructive (HOCM), 80, 81, 98, 109, 173, 236
 peripartum, 258, 259, 269
 stress or takotsubo, 293
Cardiopulmonary resuscitation (CPR), 116, 117, 123, 307
Cardioversion, 110
Carotid artery. See Artery, carotid.
Carvedilol, 121, 273
Catheter, 131–135, 172, 189–195, 205, 209, 218, 262

Catheterization, cardiac. *See* Cardiac catheterization.
Cerebrovascular accident (CVA). *See* Stroke.
Cervix, 30, 31, 38, 42, 46, 346
Chest pain, 73, 76, 99, 103, 104, 109, 113, 117–120, 127, 130, 131, 134, 136, 137, 139–141, 154, 156, 160, 170, 173, 174, 183, 189, 199, 200, 232, 234, 236, 241, 245, 248, 261, 262, 267, 270, 288, 292, 307, 319
Cholesterol, 72, 93, 94, 96, 116, 117, 155, 157, 160, 164, 180, 181, 185, 238, 245, 248, 260, 283, 285, 287, 288, 298, 299, 300, 301, 307, 309, 345, 347, 348
   cholesterol-lowering medications, 93, 155, 275, 287
   types
      high-density lipoprotein (HDL), 180–183, 283, 287, 300, 301, 309, 347, 348
      low-density lipoprotein (LDL), 180–183, 260, 283, 287, 299, 300, 301, 348
Cholestyramine, 182
Chromosomes, 28, 29, 33
Cialis, 240–243, 249, 251
Cilostazol, 93, 172
Clitoris, 31, 32, 35, 42, 44, 56, 64, 346
Clonidine, 179, 286
Clopidogrel, 87, 93, 120, 155, 174, 194, 239
Coach, 331
Coarctation of the aorta, 263
Cocaine, 313, 314, 321
Coitus. *See* Sex.
Colesevelam, 182
Colestipol, 182
Collateral(s), 73, 74, 200
Computed tomography (CT), 38, 89, 147, 167–172, 185

Congenital heart disease, 171, 262, 264, 265, 267, 268, 280
Congestive heart failure. *See* Heart failure.
Contraception. *See* Birth control.
Coping, 331
Coronary angiography. *See* Angiography, coronary.
Coronary angioplasty. *See* Angioplasty, coronary.
Coronary artery (ies)
  circumflex, 67, 346
  left anterior descending (LAD), 67, 197, 198, 346
  right (RCA), 67, 346
Coronary artery bypass graft surgery (CABG), 195–199, 217, 224, 227, 248, 290
  sex and, 224, 225, 248, 249
  women and, 290
Coronary artery disease (CAD)
  AIDS and, 319
  alcohol and, 309
  aortic stenosis and, 96
  arrhythmias and, 107, 110
  cholesterol and, 180, 181, 182
  cocaine and, 313
  coronary angiography and, 133, 134
  coronary angioplasty and, 83, 188
  coronary artery bypass graft surgery and, 195–198
  definition, 72
  diabetes and, 79
  diet and, 298, 299
  disease of other arteries and, 93
  enhanced external counterpulsation and, 199, 200
  erectile dysfunction and, 245
  evaluation of
    stress test and, 306
  evaluation of, 117, 140–142, 145, 161, 164
    computed tomography and, 169–171

magnetic resonance imaging and, 167, 171
stress test and, 148–151
heart attack and, 74
heart transplantation and, 211
high blood pressure and, 85
medications for. *See also* Tables 1 and 2, 119, 122, 173–175, 178, 182
obesity and, 303
positron-emission tomography and, 184
pregnancy and, 258, 260, 261
risk factors for, 94
sex and, 221, 226, 242, 247
tobacco and, 310, 311, 316
transmyocardial laser revascularization and, 198, 199
women and, 282–290
Coronary care unit (CCU), 117
Coronary stent. *See* Stent, coronary.
Corpus albicans, 40
Corpus cavernosum, 35
Corpus luteum, 40
Corpus spongiosum, 35
Coumadin. *See* Warfarin.
Counselor, 331, 335
C-reactive protein, 184
Creatine phosphokinase
   CPK, 128, 129, 130
   CPK-MB, 128, 129, 130
Cryptorchidism, 32
Deep vein thrombosis (DVT), 113
Defibrillator(s), 116, 118, 123, 124
Depression, 226, 232, 286, 304, 308, 324, 330, 331, 333

Diabetes, 72, 76, 79, 93, 94, 110, 117, 135, 155, 160, 161, 164, 170, 180, 193, 235, 245, 246, 248, 258, 259, 285–287, 290, 291, 294, 297, 303–307, 310, 316, 345
Diastole, 65, 80, 81, 97, 109, 132, 161–163, 200, 201
Diet(s), 155, 181, 288, 296–301, 309, 320
Digitalis. *See* digoxin.
Digoxin, 142, 176, 177, 273, 278, 286, 292, 308
Diltiazem, 107, 175, 177, 235, 236, 273
Dipyridamole, 150, 151
Dissection, 168
  aortic, 90, 91, 207, 313
  coronary, 261
Diuretics, 131, 175, 176, 238, 270, 271, 273
Divorce, 327, 329
Dobutamine, 131, 149–151
Dopamine, 58, 132
Doppler study, 143, 144, 245
Doxazosin, 179, 242
Dressler syndrome, 154
Ebstein's anomaly, 265
Echocardiogram, 142–146, 151, 153, 160, 163, 165, 168, 171, 245, 269, 278, 289, 320
  transesophageal, 144, 145, 278
  transthoracic, 143, 144, 278
Eclampsia, 260, 287
Eisenmenger's syndrome, 267
Electrocardiogram (EKG), 111, 112, 116–118, 130, 136, 137, 140–142, 148, 151, 164, 170, 178, 185, 217, 278, 288, 289, 292, 347
Electrophysiology (EP) study, 167
Embryo, 40
Enalapril, 122
Encainide, 178

Endarterectomy, 208
Endocarditis, 100–102, 204, 314, 318, 319
Endometrium, 30, 38
Enhanced external counterpulsation (EECP), 199, 200, 219
Enoxaparin, 120, 276
Enzymes, cardiac, 128, 137, 170
Ephedra, 308
Epididymis, 34
Epinephrine. *See* Adrenaline.
Eptifibatide, 193
Erectile dysfunction (ED), 232–240, 243, 245, 246, 249, 251, 315, 316, 347
Erection, 36, 37, 42, 44, 92, 232, 233, 241, 243, 244, 246, 251, 316, 347
Estrogen, 29, 40, 41, 45, 46, 47, 113, 282–284, 289
Estrous cycle, 54
Exercise, 62, 66, 67, 75, 76, 84, 116, 141, 142, 145, 147–149, 150, 151, 155, 156, 170, 181, 200, 226, 227, 228, 229, 249, 261, 267, 278, 288, 296, 297, 304–306, 315, 321
Ezetimibe, 182
Fallopian tubes, 30, 38, 39, 45, 46
Fats, 288, 299, 300
Felodipine, 175, 236, 275
Femoral artery. *See* Artery, femoral.
Fenofibrate, 183
Fertilization, 38, 40, 46, 349
Fetus, 40
Fever, 98–100, 103, 154, 291
Fiber, 181, 192, 298
Fish, 52, 299, 317
Flecainide, 178, 274
Fluoroscopy, 125, 134, 279
Fluoxetine, 233

Follicle(s), 29, 37, 38, 40
Follicle-stimulating hormone, 36, 37
Foods, 176, 298–301, 306, 308, 309
Foramen ovale, 88
Furosemide, 176
Gallop rhythm, 162
Garlic, 306, 307
Gemfibrozil, 287
Genes, 305
Genetic, 33, 53, 91, 184, 185
Gonorrhea, 55, 318, 319
Graft(s), 195–198, 207, 208, 219, 290, 294, 346
HDL. See Cholesterol, types.
Heart. See also specific topics.
  anatomy of, 62–68
  artificial (mechanical), 211
Heart attack, 78
  arrhythmias and, 123–127
  cardiac enzymes and, 128–130
  causes, 75, 91, 94
  complications of, 97, 151–154
  coronary angiography and, 134–136
  definition of, 74
  diabetics and, 79
  evaluation of, 116, 127, 140, 156
  sex and, 75, 76, 242, 248–250
  silent, 76
  ST-elevation myocardial infarction, 118, 133, 135, 188
  symptoms, 76, 77
  treatment, 117–122, 131–133, 154, 155
Heart block, 105

Heart failure, 77–85, 93–99, 114, 122, 127, 131, 143, 152, 160–164, 173–180, 185, 200, 233, 236–239, 242, 249, 250, 258, 262, 263, 266, 268–270, 280, 289, 291, 292, 301, 318–321
Heart transplantation. See Transplant, heart.
Hemoglobin, 63
Heparin, 120, 133, 193, 276, 277
Herbal preparations, 308
High blood pressure. See Hypertension.
High-density lipoprotein (HDL). See Cholesterol, types.
Hobbies, 334
Holter monitor, 165, 166, 268, 278
Homocysteine, 184
Hormone replacement therapy, 41, 283–285
Human immunodeficiency virus (HIV). See Acquired immune deficiency syndrome (AIDS).
Hormones, 28–32, 35, 36, 40, 41, 47, 57, 58, 83, 243, 283–285, 328, 332, 347–350
Hydralazine, 179, 180, 271
Hydrochlorothiazide, 175, 238, 273
Hymen, 31
Hypertension, 84, 85, 93, 96, 100, 110, 160, 161, 173–175, 179, 180, 181, 200, 233, 234, 238, 245, 248, 259, 262–268, 285, 290, 291, 301, 310, 316
Hyperthyroidism, 83, 107, 108, 164
Hypertrophic obstructive cardiomyopathy. See Cardiomyopathy, hypertrophic obstructive (HOCM).
Hypotension, orthostatic, 179
Illegal drugs, 312–314
Implantable cardioverter-defibrillator, 223
Impotence, 233, 238 See also Erectile dysfunction.
Infarction. See Myocardial infarction.

Infection(s), 31, 79, 83, 91, 96, 98, 100–103, 114, 128, 145, 210, 211, 215, 263, 268, 314, 318, 319, 325
INR, 203
Insertable loop recorder, 166
Intensive Care Unit (ICU), 117, 131, 311
Intercourse. See Sex.
Intimacy, 59, 60, 221, 328
Intra-aortic balloon pump, 132
Introitus, 31, 43
Irbesartan, 122, 274
Ischemia. See Myocardial ischemia.
Isosorbide, 240, 241, 273
Kidney(s), 61, 82, 85, 89, 168, 172
Kielcolt-Glaser, Dr. Janice, 330
Labetolol, 179
Lactation. See Breastfeeding.
Laser, 191, 198, 199, 208, 219
Laughter, 332, 333, 336
LDL. See Cholesterol, types.
Left atrium, 62–65, 68, 81, 88, 97, 99, 100, 102, 104, 109, 110, 143, 201, 205, 206, 209, 212, 262, 348
Left ventricle, 62–68, 78–83, 88, 97–99, 103, 104, 108–110, 131, 132, 135, 143–149, 152–154, 162, 164, 199, 200, 201, 205, 212, 213, 216, 236, 263–266, 292, 293, 345, 348
Legumes, 299
Levitra, 240–243, 249, 251
Libido, 234, 238
Lidocaine, 126, 177
Lipoprotein. See Cholesterol.
Lisinopril, 122, 274
Liver, 61, 64, 127, 155, 164, 182, 309, 314
Low-density lipoprotein (LDL). See Cholesterol, types.

Lovastatin, 182, 307
Love, 58–60, 316, 328, 333
  biochemistry of, 58
  expression of, 59
  sex and, 59
Lung(s), 54, 61–64, 68, 81, 82, 113, 114, 126–128, 131, 141, 143, 146, 149, 161, 164, 262, 265, 267, 285, 288, 310, 319, 349, 350
Luteinizing hormone, 36, 38
Lymphoma, 319
Magnesium, 176, 301
Magnetic resonance imaging (MRI), 89, 167–172, 185
Markusic, Dr. James, 58, 59
Marriage, 58, 327–330, 333, 335
Master's two-step test, 140
Maze procedure, 218
Medications. *See* Table 2. *See* under specific name.
Menopause, 30, 41, 42, 257, 282–287
Metabolic equivalent (MET), 247, 249
Metastasis, 102
Methyldopa, 179, 238, 273
Metoprolol, 121, 234, 273, 278
Mexilitene, 177
Miller, Dr. Michael, 332
Mitral regurgitation, 97–100, 133, 135, 157, 162, 175, 237, 238, 270
Mitral stenosis, 99, 100, 103, 108–110, 143, 144, 164, 174, 205, 206, 267-271
Mitral valve
  function of, 62, 65
Mitral valve prolapse, 97, 164, 288, 291
Mittelschmerz, 38
Monitor. *See also* Holter monitor.
  event, 165, 166, 268
Morphine, 118

Murmur(s), 153, 163
Myocardial infarction (MI), 74, 116, 118, 130, 133, 135, 188, 221 See also Heart attack.
Myocardial ischemia, 73, 74, 94, 140, 249
Myocardial perfusion imaging (MPI), 142, 146–151, 168, 184, 278, 289, 348
Myocarditis, 79, 212, 268, 318, 319
Myocardium, 72, 83, 133
Myoglobin, 128–130
Myxoma, 102, 103
Nadolol, 273
Natural selection, 53
Nervous system
  parasympathetic, and sex, 43, 246
  sympathetic, and sex, 44, 246
Niacin, 183, 275
Nicardipine, 175, 273
Niemark, Jill, 332
Nifedipine, 175, 236, 273
Nitrates, 174, 180, 240, 241, 242, 249, 273
Nitroglycerin, 116, 117, 119, 131, 154, 157, 174, 239, 241, 273
Nitroprusside, 131
Nocturnal emission, 37, 233
Nocturnal penile tumescence testing, 233
Norepinephrine, 58, 132
Nutrition, 255
Nuts, 299
Obesity, 248, 303
Olmesartan, 274
Omega-3 fatty acids, 299, 307, 308
Oocyte, 29
Ophthalmoscope, 161
Orgasm, 44, 45, 55–57, 60, 247, 286, 315, 316
Ovaries, 29, 32, 36, 37, 41, 47, 347, 350

Ovum, 29, 37–40, 46, 347
Oxygen, 30, 63, 64, 67, 68, 72, 73, 83, 93, 94, 113, 116, 118, 119, 121, 128, 196, 226, 247, 261, 263, 265, 345, 350
Oxytocin, 57, 60, 331
Ozarks Marriage Matters (OMM), 330
Pacemaker, 223, 349
  external transthoracic, 124–126
  malfunction, 215, 216
  permanent, 124, 213, 214
  temporary transvenous, 124, 125, 131, 167, 213
Paclitaxel, 194
Paroxetine, 233
Paroxysmal supraventricular tachycardia (PSVT), 111, 269
Patent ductus arteriosus (PDA), 209
Patent foramen ovale (PFO), 88
Penile fracture, 43
Penile implant, 244
Penis, 31, 35, 36, 42–47, 63, 64, 92, 232–235, 241, 243–246, 302, 316, 318, 323, 324, 349–351
Pericardial effusion, 103, 143, 319, 320
Pericardial tamponade, 103
Pericarditis, 103, 164
  constrictive, 103
Pericardium, 99, 103, 104, 114, 152, 154, 203
Peripheral arterial disease, 92, 93, 200, 201, 245, 248, 250, 290, 310
Phenylethylamine (PEA), 58
Placenta, 30
Plaque. See Atherosclerosis.
Positive psychology, 331, 333
Positron-emission tomography (PET), 56, 184, 186
Post, Dr. Stephen, 331, 332
Potassium, 107, 112, 122, 155, 164, 176, 301

Pravastatin, 182
Prayer, 324, 325–327
Prazosin, 179
Preeclampsia, 259, 260, 287
Pregnancy, 29, 30, 39–41, 45–48, 58, 113, 254–280, 287, 349, 351
  arrhythmias and, 256, 268, 269
  congenital heart disease and, 262–267
  coronary artery disease and, 260, 261
  hypertension and, 259, 260
  medications and, 272, 273, 274, 275, 276
  myocarditis and, 268
  valve disease and, 269, 270
Premature atrial contraction (PAC), 106–108, 256, 268
Premature ventricular contraction (PVC), 106, 107, 256, 268
Princeton guidelines, 248–250
Procainamide, 126, 178, 242, 274
Progesterone, 29, 30, 40, 41, 47, 283
Propafenone, 178, 274
Propranolol, 121, 234, 272, 273
Prostate, 35, 102, 179, 242, 246
Protein, 259
Pseudoaneurysm, 152–154
Pseudoephedrine, 107
Psychologist(s), 331, 335
PTCA (percutaneous transluminal coronary angioplasty). *See* Angioplasty, coronary.
Puberty, 30, 36, 37, 264, 347, 350
Pulmonary artery, 62, 64, 65, 113, 131, 209, 263, 264, 266, 349
Pulmonary edema, 131
Pulmonary embolism, 113

Pulmonary hypertension, 265–268, 280, 319
  primary, 267
Pulmonary veins, 64
Pulmonic valve, 349
  endocarditis and, 100, 314
  function of, 62, 65
  regurgitation, 100
  stenosis, 262
Quinidine, 178, 242, 274
Radiation, 103, 142, 168, 195, 258, 261, 278–280
Radioactive material, 146, 148, 156, 195, 348
Ranolazine, 177
Regurgitation, aortic. See Aortic regurgitation.
Regurgitation, mitral. See Mitral regurgitation.
Rehabilitation, cardiac, 156, 226, 229, 296, 330
Rejection, 210, 211
Renal. See Kidney.
Restenosis, 193, 194, 195
Reteplase, 133
Rhabdomyoma, 103
Rhabdomyosarcoma, 103
Rheumatic fever, 98–100, 257, 269, 270, 291
Rhythm
  birth control, 45
  heart, 77, 80, 81, 98, 99, 105, 107, 111, 114, 123, 124, 130, 137, 151, 154, 164–166, 216–219, 221, 223, 225, 233, 236, 238, 274, 291, 313, 314, 345, 347, 350, 351
Right atrium, 62–68, 81, 88, 104, 125, 205, 209, 214–217, 262, 350
Right ventricle, 62–68, 78, 81, 103, 104, 113, 124–126, 131, 149, 152, 162, 211, 212, 214, 216, 217, 264–266, 319, 349, 350
Risk factors
  for aortic stenosis, 96

for carotid and arterial disease, 93
for coronary artery disease, 160, 310
   in women, 258, 282, 285, 286
for heart disease, 76, 258
Ross procedure, 204
Rosuvastatin, 182
S_1, S_2, 161, 162
S_3, S_4, 162
Saphenous vein, 196, 224
Scrotum, 32–34, 244
Sedative(s), 124, 233
Seldinger technique, 125, 134
Selective serotonin reuptake inhibitors (SSRI), 233
Semen, 31, 35, 38, 44, 45
Seminal vesicles, 34, 35
Sex, 23–32, 35–37, 41–48, 51–62, 75, 76, 94, 156, 214, 218–229, 232, 234, 237–239, 242–251, 254, 286, 296, 298, 302, 306, 314–318, 321, 333, 335, 347, 349, 350, 351
   alcohol and, 315
   biological purpose of, 52, 53
   coronary angiography and, 222
   features of human sexuality, 54, 55, 58, 59
   gender, 36, 52, 170, 249
   health and, 314, 315, 328, 335
   heart attack and, 75, 226, 248, 249
   heart disease and, 221
   heart rate and blood pressure during, 246, 247
   heart surgery and, 225
   obesity and, 302
   pacemaker and, 223
   risk of, 248–250
   tobacco and, 316
Sexually transmitted diseases (STD), 55, 318, 319
Sildenafil. *See* Viagra.

Simvastatin, 182, 275
Sinus node, 66, 77, 105, 106, 107
Sirolimus, 194
Smirnoff, Yakov, 333
Smoking. *See* Tobacco.
Sodium, 164, 301
Sotalol, 178, 242
Spermatozoa. *See* Sperm cells.
Sperm cells, 32–47, 316, 334, 347, 349, 350
Spironolactone, 175, 286
St. John's wort, 308
Statin(s), 157, 181–183, 275, 278, 286, 287, 307
Stem cells, 184
Stenosis, aortic. See Aortic stenosis.
Stenosis, mitral. See Mitral stenosis.
Stent
  coronary, 193, 194, 346
  other arteries, 208
Sternotomy, 196, 198, 199, 225
Sternum, 62, 196, 198, 225
Streptokinase, 133
Stress, 227, 232, 247, 250, 255, 288, 292, 304
Stress test
  exercise, 149, 156, 170, 227, 249, 288, 306
  pharmacologic, 149–151, 171, 184
  screening for heart disease, 306
  sex and, 227, 248, 249, 250
  women and, 288, 289
    in pregnancy, 261, 278
Stroke, 85–88, 91, 100, 101, 103, 110, 135, 153, 171, 174, 182, 206, 232, 239, 242, 245–250, 259, 264, 267, 275, 284, 285, 289, 290, 294, 308, 310, 319
Supplements, nutritional, 306–308
Support groups, 304, 331

Supraventricular tachycardia, 108, 111, 173, 218, 236, 269, 291
Swan-Ganz catheter, 131
Syncope, 82, 166, 255, 270
Syphilis, 55, 91, 317, 318, 319
Systole, 65, 132, 148, 149, 161, 163, 200, 201
Tachycardia, 77, 108, 111, 112, 126, 127, 216, 217, 291, 351
Technetium-99m, 146–149, 184
  sestamibi, 146–148
  tetrofosmin, 146–148
Telemetry, 130
Tenecteplase, 133
Terazosin, 179, 242
Testis (testes), 32–36, 47, 316, 350
Testosterone, 28, 29, 32, 33, 36, 41, 47, 243, 350
Tetralogy of Fallot, 264, 265
Thallium-201, 146–148, 184
Thiazide, 175, 238
Thrombolytics, 129, 133–136
Thrombus, 88
Thyroid, 83, 105, 107, 108, 127, 164, 256, 268, 272, 274, 304
Ticlopidine, 174, 239
Tilt table test, 166
Tobacco, 93, 160, 233, 310, 311, 313, 315–317, 321
Tocainide, 177, 178
TOPS, 304
Torsades de pointes, 108, 112
Torsemide, 176
Transient ischemic attack (TIA), 87, 88
Transmyocardial laser revascularization (TMLR), 198, 199
Transplant, heart, 83, 210, 211, 212, 228, 258, 268
Transposition of the great vessels, 264, 265

Tricuspid valve
  Ebstein's anomaly and, 265
  endocarditis and, 100, 314
  function of, 62, 65, 350
  regurgitation, 265
  stenosis, 100
Triglycerides, 180–183, 260, 283, 287, 298, 299, 301, 307
Troponin, 128–130
Tuberculosis, 103
Tumors, 85, 102, 103, 114, 143, 171
Twiddler's syndrome, 215
Ultrasound, ultrasonography, 192, 332
Umbilical cord, 30, 349
Urethra, 31, 35, 44, 243, 318, 346
Uterus, 30, 31, 38, 39, 40, 46, 57, 256, 257, 283, 346, 347, 349
Vacuum device, 243, 244
Vagina, 31, 32, 38, 40, 42–47, 63, 64, 346, 349
Valve(s). *See* Aortic valve; Mitral valve; Pulmonic valve; Tricuspid valve.
Valves, artificial
  bioprosthetic, 201, 203, 204, 271
  mechanical, 201–204, 271
  pregnancy and, 271
  warfarin and, 202–204, 239, 271
Valvotomy, 205–207, 219, 262, 270
Vardenafil. *See* Levitra.
Vas deferens, 34, 35, 45
Vegetations, 88, 101, 144
Vein, 30, 88, 113, 124, 125, 127, 131, 134, 146, 147, 150, 167, 170, 176, 196, 197, 205, 208, 211, 214, 218, 224, 256, 313, 314, 348
Ventricular assist device (VAD), 212

Ventricular fibrillation (VF), 77, 79, 108, 116, 123, 126, 127, 216, 217
Ventricular septal defect
congenital, 104, 264, 266
myocardial infarction and, 152, 153
Ventricular tachycardia (VT), 77, 79, 108, 112, 123, 126, 127, 154, 167, 177, 216–218, 291
Verapamil, 107, 175, 177, 235, 273, 308
Viagra, 240–243, 246, 249, 251, 286
Viets, Elaine, 334
Vitamins, 298, 306, 308
vitamin K, 202
Volunteering, 332
Warfarin, 87, 93, 174, 202–204, 239, 244, 271, 272, 275–278
warfarin embryopathy, 275
Wedge pressure, 131
Weight loss, 298, 300, 304, 308
Wet dream, 37
Withering, Dr. William, 176
Womb. *See* Uterus.
X-ray, 142, 168, 169, 208
chest, 116–118, 161, 164, 185, 278, 279
Zygote, 39

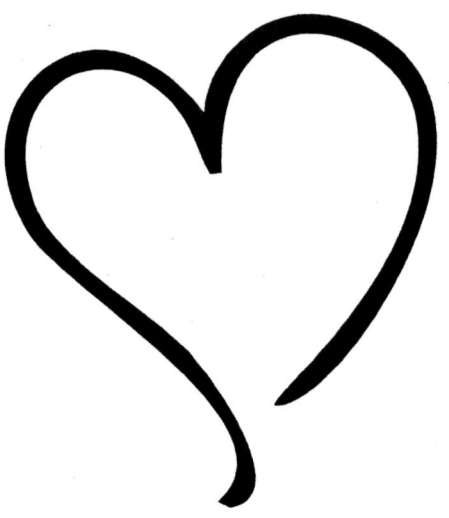